Thrive at Any Weight

Thrive at Any Weight

Eating to Nourish Body, Soul, and Self-Esteem

Nancy Ellis-Ordway

Foreword by Harriet Brown

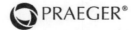

PRAEGER®

An Imprint of ABC-CLIO, LLC
Santa Barbara, California • Denver, Colorado

Library of Congress Cataloging in Publication Control Number: 2019945443

ISBN: 978-1-4408-7023-1 (print)
        978-1-4408-7024-8 (ebook)

23 22 21 20 19   1 2 3 4 5

This book is also available as an eBook.

Praeger
An Imprint of ABC-CLIO, LLC

ABC-CLIO, LLC
147 Castilian Drive
Santa Barbara, California 93117
www.abc-clio.com

This book is printed on acid-free paper (∞)

Manufactured in the United States of America

To my husband,
Frederick Stephen Ordway,
who taught me to believe in myself

Contents

Foreword

Not long ago I gave a talk to a group of pediatricians. The subject was anorexia and specifically how pediatricians could and should screen more aggressively for the disease. I presented them with research on how outcomes improved with early diagnosis and treatment and suggested the importance of tracking adolescent growth curves to make sure teens were not losing weight or—harder to notice—failing to gain weight as they grew. It was a subject that resonated deeply with me because it had happened to my own daughter, who was diagnosed with anorexia at age 14.

I will never forget the 50-something male doctor in the front row who sat, arms folded, and glared—there's no other word for it—the whole time I was speaking. During the Q and A, he was the first to raise his hand.

"Do you know how many obese kids I see?" he challenged. "I'm way more worried about type 2 diabetes than anorexia. A little weight loss would be good for most of them."

I wish I could say his attitude was unusual. I have encountered it repeatedly from not just pediatricians but all sorts of medical professionals who are deeply invested in the idea that fatness is the worst thing that can happen to a person. As a culture, we conflate thinness with not just beauty and good health but goodness itself. We equate thinness with virtue, righteousness, and morality.

At the height of my daughter's illness, when she was gaunt and hollow-eyed and sad, she routinely got compliments on her body. Acquaintances who found out she was sick would say, self-deprecatingly, "I could use a little anorexia myself!" A saleswoman in a clothing store, where I was trying on clothes, once said to her, "Aren't you lucky—you got the thin genes!" The lab tech doing her EKG on the day she was diagnosed asked her for diet tips.

I was horrified by these kinds of comments. Does everyone in the United States have body dysmorphia? Can we not see the difference between healthy and sick, between thin and skeletal? My daughter was not a model; she was visibly dying.

Humans are social animals. We are always trying to figure out where we stand in relation to the rest of the group. And part of how we do that is by internalizing the group's rules and customs. I cannot fault any of us for buying into the cultural norms around weight and body image because we all drink the fatphobic Kool-Aid every day. *Of course* it affects us. Of course we are confused. Of course we have distorted ideas of what we should weigh, what we should look like, and what we should and should not eat.

And all of that is why Nancy Ellis-Ordway's book is so important. With great care, she explores and deconstructs not just myths around food, eating, and weight but also the dysfunctional thought patterns that have taken root in so many of us. She questions some of our most deeply held beliefs and shines a light on the ways our thinking about food, eating, and weight hold us back from living fully.

One of the things I value most about this book is Ellis-Ordway's perspective as a therapist who treats eating disorders. Too often, clinical conversations around weight and weight stigma, on the one hand, and eating disorders on the other happen in separate universes, as the comment from the angry pediatrician suggests. But, of course, they are connected, as are the clinicians who see patients across the weight spectrum.

More than once, I have heard therapists and other professionals tell patients with anorexia or bulimia, "Don't worry, we'll make sure you don't gain too much weight during treatment." This is exactly what someone with an eating disorder wants to hear. But this attitude is not just fundamentally antithetical to the goal of treatment, which is to bring about full recovery; it is also fatphobic. It reinforces the idea that fat is bad and that becoming fatter (whatever that might mean for any specific patient) is something to be mitigated or, better yet, avoided. There is no way a treatment provider with this attitude can be effective.

These attitudes affect all of us, whether we have eating disorders, treat them, or are just struggling to figure out how to take care of ourselves in a world of distorted views on weight and body image. Ellis-Ordway's thought-provoking questions will make you see things differently. For instance, writing about the common diet advice "Don't eat when you're not hungry," she asks, "First of all, how do you define hunger? Does your stomach have to rumble? Do you have to be lightheaded? Are you hungry enough to justify eating without shame?" Considering these questions will help you understand your own hunger and fullness cues and make choices based on what is good for you rather than on generic (and misguided) advice.

Another one of Ellis-Ordway's main takeaways is that despite what we are constantly told by medical professions, by media, and by friends and family, weight and eating issues are not just matters of personal responsibility. They are part of a bigger picture of stigma and oppression that affects us all, no matter how much we weigh or what our bodies look like. "Learning to accept and appreciate our bodies is challenging in a culture where some people make money from stealing our self-esteem so that they can sell it back to us at a profit," she writes (chapter 5). No kidding! This fact seems self-evident once it is pointed out, but it is awfully hard to believe when you are deep in self-loathing and self-doubt.

And that is the greatest gift of Nancy Ellis-Ordway's book. In clear, accessible language, she explains many of the conundrums that baffle and constrict us, and she gives us the information and tools to free ourselves. In writing about issues like weight bias, healthism, privilege, food insecurity, stereotypes, and more, she calls out social paradoxes and empowers us to advocate for ourselves with doctors. She gives practical information on how to talk to our children about food and body image. Most important, she helps us figure out how to thrive in a world that sometimes seems to have gone mad when it comes to the relentless pursuit of thinness at any cost.

Harriet Brown

Preface

If you kept changing the way people see the world, you ended up changing the way you saw yourself.[1]

About Me

Too many people have a broken relationship with food, and it is ruining their lives. This fact is dreadful, heartbreaking, and totally unnecessary. It is a situation that can be changed, and I am committed to doing what I can to change it. The path that led me to this place, personally and professionally, started with William Bennett and Joel Gurin's *The Dieter's Dilemma* in 1985.[2]

I grew up skinny in the late 1950s and early 1960s, when the accepted standard of beauty was curvy and voluptuous. Cleavage, of which I had none, was highly valued. I had my fair share of body discontent and unhappiness, but I was oblivious to anti-fat stigma that was already being internalized by my larger-bodied friends. Weight Watchers was just getting started, sugar-free soda tasted nasty and was only for people with diabetes, and mealtime always included dessert. I had no idea how much I was benefiting from "thin privilege." It certainly never occurred to me that it was something I could lose.

My body did not instantly revert to its prepregnancy weight after my first child was born, but by then I knew better than to go on a diet. When my waistline disappeared shortly after my 40th birthday (as it does for many women), I knew better than to go on a diet. When menopause added more curves, I knew better than to go on a diet. I knew that dieting would make things worse. *The Dieter's Dilemma* saved me from decades of dieting, weight cycling, and body dissatisfaction. I have been able to tolerate the changes that age has made to my body without trying to interfere. I consider it a great blessing that I knew better.

I have always been fascinated by the way people use food for more than fueling their bodies: to soothe, to comfort, to celebrate, to affirm, or to establish identity. As a freshman in college, I noticed all the stories that my classmates told about the food customs in their families of origin and how often they labeled them as, "We do this because we are Italian/German/Irish/fill-in-the-blank." They might be describing very similar traditions, but it was clear that food was closely connected to identity, belonging, and acceptance. It only made sense for me to study nutrition, foods, and family relationships.

Some years back, I taught Introduction to Social Work at a local college. I started by explaining my belief that career success can be tied to finding an option that is based on whatever activity you most often got into trouble for as a child. I most often got into trouble for sticking my nose in other people's business. Now I make a living from doing that very thing. In fact, I have a degree in sticking my nose in other people's business and have a license to do so.

Combining an undergraduate degree in home economics (now known as family and consumer sciences) with a graduate degree in social work led me to a position with the Anorexia Bulimia Treatment and Education Center (ABtec) at St. John's Mercy Medical Center in St. Louis, Missouri. As part of my orientation, the medical director handed me a copy of *The Dieter's Dilemma*, and I soon realized that much of what I thought I knew was wrong. That book changed the personal and professional trajectory of my life.

Working at ABtec changed my worldview. For those with eating disorders, food is not about nutrition or belonging, and it is certainly not about celebration or joy. For them, the act of eating is terrifying, and their relationship with food is one of anguish. Recovery from an eating disorder is excruciatingly difficult and requires great courage and perseverance. I became aware that beyond those who found their way into treatment with us, there were countless more in the world who struggled with various levels of discomfort around food, eating, and their bodies, and they did not even realize there was any other way to be. Somehow, in our culture, having a broken relationship with food and eating has become accepted as the norm. I am compelled to push back against that.

Dying is not the only outcome of having an eating disorder; it is just the most dramatic. A disordered relationship with food limits possibilities, impairs quality of life, and steals joy.

It has been my great privilege to continue working in the eating disorder treatment field. I have been honored by the many individuals and families who have shared their stories and struggles with me. Over time, it became clear that the problems of disordered eating are firmly rooted in weight stigma and unrealistic values around appearance. Addressing these issues, on individual and societal levels, is my lifelong passion.

One of the challenges of working in the health field, especially mental health, is translating the knowledge that comes from research and academic study into information that can be used in therapy and applied in everyday life. This has been a large focus of my work for many years, and this book is an attempt to share it all.

I recently had lunch with a friend who is new to the Health At Every Size (HAES) concept. She had questions, and I enjoyed talking about one of my favorite topics. Then she asked something that brought me up short and shifted my perspective. She asked, "Did you discover HAES in time to not pass on body insecurities to your children?" Yes. Yes, I did. I was in the right place at the right time to learn. It was a gift of grace, and I want to share it. I want more people to discover this new way of thinking, of living, and of decreasing individual and intergenerational body insecurity. And so I wrote this book.

Acknowledgments

Writing a book is not a solitary undertaking; I have many folks to thank. Finding a supportive community in a world that focuses on weight loss has become easier with social media. Special thanks go to Dr. Claudia Clark, who introduced me to the Showmethedata email listserv, which was a precursor to the Association for Size Diversity and Health. I could not have done this without all of you in those groups. A special shout-out goes to Dr. Angela Meadows, who has broadened my horizons and taught me how to organize myself to write. Sitting next to you at lunch that day at the conference was one of the best decisions I ever made.

I have the great good fortune to have a large number of assorted in-laws who have supported me in this journey. In addition, Megan, Mary Jo, Erica, and Jen at the Yoga Studio of Jefferson City have also made immeasurable contributions to maintaining my balance and my mental health.

I am grateful to those who love me enough to proofread the manuscript and provide feedback: Candie Hill, Dana Schuster, and my favorite son, Stephen Ordway.

My children and children-in-law, Ellie Ordway-West, Stephen Ordway, Josh West, and Dawn King, have been never-ending sources of encouragement, motivation, suggestions, food, love, and perspective. And last, but certainly not least, I owe a huge thank-you to my wonderful husband, Fred Ordway, who accepts and supports me in all my various moods.

Most of all, I am grateful to the many individuals who have allowed me to be part of their life journeys by trusting me and working with me in therapy. Thank you for letting me walk along the path of healing with you. I have learned so much in the process!

About the Cover

In August 2018, I was a coleader for a preconference workshop for the Association for Size Diversity and Health's annual conference in Portland, Oregon. After most of us had left for the airport on the last day, several people, including two of my copresenters, participated in a photo shoot in which they smashed scales. I am delighted that one of those photos graces the cover of this book. To see more of the work of this talented photographer, S. Lindley Ashline, go to lindleyashline.com.

CHAPTER ONE

Where Are We, and How Did We Get Here?

Dieting is dangerous. The pursuit of weight loss, whether you call it a diet, a lifestyle change, portion control, or "making better choices," is hazardous to our physical, mental, emotional, and financial well-being. This is a shocking statement. Many people think that even making this statement is dangerous and risky, but there is an expanding awareness that our cultural beliefs and attitudes about weight, eating, and well-being urgently need to be reevaluated.

How did this topic become so complicated and contentious? And what can we do about it?

Newspapers are filled with headlines about the "Obesity Epidemic," and bookstores are filled with books that claim to help people lose weight. Grocery stores are filled with low-cal, low-carb, low-fat foods, yet people just seem to be getting fatter. Everyone agrees that there is a problem, a big problem, but none of the many solutions suggested seem to work.

Perhaps we have been going about it all wrong.

I am a psychotherapist trained in several different theories of counseling, and I have been working with people who have eating, weight, and body image problems for more than three decades. I have researched behavioral approaches to weight loss, and I have worked on an inpatient psychiatric unit dedicated to treating people with anorexia and bulimia nervosa. I have attended and presented at several national conferences that focused not only on these life-threatening illnesses but also such related issues as obesity, nutrition, cultural influences, binge eating, body image distortion, and weight stigma, especially as they are related to depression, anxiety, and low self-esteem.

It is clear to me that the cultural preoccupation with weight and weight loss, the focus on the dangers of higher weights, and the distaste and stigma directed at larger bodies have resulted in body dissatisfaction and shame in countless individuals. The pathology seen in eating disorders is deeply rooted in the cultural antipathy directed toward anyone who is not slender. The toxic effects of weight stigma are so interwoven into the fabric of our culture that most people do not notice, even as they are affected by it.

The epidemic of weight stigma gets much less attention than the so-called "Obesity Epidemic" in the media, but an increasing number of researchers, treatment clinicians, and activists are identifying the negative cultural attitudes about large bodies as harmful to individual and public health. Large people are treated badly in public places, online, at work, and in intimate settings with those who love them. The prevailing attitude is that if they feel badly enough about themselves, they will change. Meanwhile, those who are slender are terrified that they might gain weight and also be treated as badly. Weight stigma leads to anxiety, body shame, and disordered eating across the spectrum of body sizes. "Thin privilege" protects one from overt discrimination, but it does not protect one from internalizing the effects of weight stigma.

Body shame is rampant. I continue to treat individuals with anorexia and bulimia nervosa in a private practice setting, but I also see individuals with a wide range of eating and body image problems, who do not fit neatly into a diagnostic category. By combining information about nutrition, body acceptance, the science of weight, and cultural pressures, I am able to offer my patients an approach that they find helpful and very different from anything they have found elsewhere. This is what I hope to share with you, the reader.

A major challenge in writing a book like this is deciding where to start and how to organize the information. In chapter 1, I will focus on some foundational background material. Chapter 2 is the "sciencey" part, which some readers may find overly technical. However, from teaching workshops and having conversations about this topic, I have found that I need to start with credible, legitimate, and evidence-based information to counter the misinformation that pervades our societal ideas about food, eating, weight, and health before addressing what to do about it. If you feel like you already know enough about these topics, feel free to skip chapter 2 or leave it for later. Chapter 3 offers ways to change your thinking about how you eat by embracing an internal locus of control and by considering the message you give yourself about your own worth in the way you eat. Chapter 4 provides specific, concrete suggestions and ideas for revamping or overhauling your relationship with food and eating. In chapter 5, I suggest ways to improve attitudes and beliefs about body image and movement. Chapters 6 and 7 tackle the issue of weight stigma, first on a personal level and then with a focus on systemic cultural aspects. Chapter 7 addresses social justice and social determinants of health in the context of weight stigma.

Interacting with medical professionals is often challenging for those with body image concerns, so chapter 8 offers ideas on ways to negotiate trips to the doctor. Chapter 9 is centered on children. This section is not just for parents. All of us interact with children, at least occasionally; therefore, it is important to understand how body image pressures affect young folks. In chapter 10, I present some suggestions for continuing to incorporate these ideas into your life as well as suggestions for further reading. Final thoughts make up chapter 11. Chapters 2, 7, and 9 focus on information and have a lot of references. The other chapters are more personal and include specific suggestions for change. I have tried to achieve a reasonable order of presentation, but, of course, you may read the chapters in any order you choose.

Stories do a better job of explaining ideas than facts and statistics, so I have shared stories throughout to illustrate important points. All the names have been changed to maintain confidentiality, and, in some cases, similar stories have been combined.

On a side note, I love to read. I have collected and included quotes from sources that may or may not be related to this topic because they illustrate points that I want to make. For specific reading suggestions, see chapter 10.

Men May Be from Mars and Women from Venus, but We All Eat at the Same Buffet on Earth

The vast majority of books, programs, and research about food and eating issues focus on women. There are cultural reasons for this, but the fact remains that men sometimes get shortchanged. Most of my counseling experience has been with women, and women are more likely to struggle with these issues and to talk to one another about them. There certainly are men (and boys) in the world whose lives are significantly constrained by food and weight issues, but there are fewer resources for them. I apologize that this book is focused more on women's experiences, but I hope that it will be of help to people of all genders.

I also realize that not everyone fits neatly into a binary gender category. As a culture, we have not agreed on a standard convention for pronouns; therefore, I have chosen to be old-fashioned and have used singular, binary pronouns throughout the book.

I try to be aware that I am writing from a position of privilege. For many individuals, the negative effects of weight stigma are compounded by racial, heteronormative, cisgender, ableist, and other intersectional biases. It is beyond my ability to address all these, and I apologize for that in advance.

A Few Words about Words

Originally, the word *diet* referred to whatever was normally consumed by an organism to acquire energy. In our culture, it sometimes means a particular way of eating to manage a specific medical condition, such as a "diabetic diet" or a "gluten-free diet," but generally it has come to mean the deliberate restriction of intake for the purpose of losing weight. It is this last definition that I will use throughout this book.

"Eating disorder" refers to one of several clinical conditions as defined by the *Diagnostic and Statistical Manual of Mental Disorders* (DSM) published by the American Psychiatric Association (APA).[1] These definitions have changed over time, through several updates of the manual.

The term *anorexia* literally means a loss of appetite. It is often used in medical records to refer to a loss of appetite caused by one or more of a variety of reasons, such as a side effect from medication, from a medical condition, or as a result of chemotherapy. The term *anorexia nervosa* was coined in 1873 by a physician in England, Sir William Gull, who was treating a young woman who was "wasting away." He called it "a loss of appetite due to nerves." This is inaccurate, because sufferers of the clinical condition of anorexia nervosa do not lose their appetites; rather, they deny their hunger in a relentless pursuit of thinness. We are, however, still stuck with the name more than a century later.

When eating disorders began to attract more attention from treatment professionals, some patients described, in addition to very restrictive eating, a pattern of binging and purging. The term used for this was "bulimia," which means "ox hunger." Since the term bulimia referred to binge eating, some people began to use it to mean excessive eating without purging, which meant there still was no specific term for the pattern of binging and purging. For a while, this pattern was referred to as "bulimarexia" (because what we really needed was yet another word that nobody could pronounce, and certainly nobody could spell). This term can still occasionally be found in books and publications written before the APA codified the definitions into distinct types.[2] The 2013 revision of the *Diagnostic and Statistical Manual of Mental Disorders* (DSM-5) includes the following categories:

Anorexia Nervosa: This includes a refusal to maintain a minimally normal weight, intense fear of gaining weight, body image disturbance, and, in women, loss of menstrual periods. Anorexia nervosa is further separated into restricting type and binge-eating/purging type. Low body weight is required for this diagnosis.

Bulimia Nervosa: This is characterized by recurrent episodes of binge eating in which a large amount of food is consumed and the person has a sense of loss of control. The episodes are followed by recurrent compensatory behaviors, such as self-induced vomiting, misuse of laxatives or diuretics, fasting, and excessive exercise, and a self-evaluation unduly influenced by body shape and weight. Bulimia nervosa is further categorized as purging and non-purging type, depending on the compensatory behavior used. Body weight may be average or high.

Binge Eating Disorder: This describes recurrent episodes of eating large amounts of food while feeling out of control, followed by feelings of distress, shame, and guilt. The DSM-5 specifically excludes being overweight or obese as a criteria. People with binge eating disorder come in all sizes.

Other Specified Feeding or Eating Disorder includes situations where most but not all criteria are met for one of the other categories. For instance, a woman meets all the criteria for anorexia nervosa except that she still has periods. It also includes night eating syndrome and purging without binging.[3]

The DSM-5, for the first time, specifically describes "atypical anorexia," which means all the behaviors of anorexia nervosa are present, but the person is not considered "underweight." It is quite possible for an individual to have all of the symptoms of anorexia nervosa without being considered underweight, especially if the person started at a weight considered "obese." He may be at a weight that is too low for him as an individual but with many or all the medical complications associated with low weight. People with atypical anorexia often have difficulty accessing adequate care, because medical professionals may believe that only very underweight people need treatment, or their health insurance carrier may refuse to cover treatment because they do not meet the criteria of having a low body mass index (BMI). Eating disorder symptoms can wreck a person's life, regardless of actual weight.

Each of these categories has an assigned code number. Insurance companies do not like to cover treatment unless they have a specific, acceptable code number for the problem, regardless of how much havoc it may be wreaking in someone's life. Accurate diagnostic labels are usually necessary to access insurance payment for treatment.

The term *body image* is used differently by different people. Rita Freedman defines it as "a complex combination of attitudes, feelings and values."[4] It is not solely, or even primarily, based on appearance. It includes how we think about ourselves and our bodies, how we feel about our bodies, how well we function, and what kinds of physical experiences we have had. It is influenced by history, the media, our culture, our families, aging, illness, and a host of other things. When I use the term *body image*, I am referring to this very complex concept.

Overweight, *obese*, and *fat* are all words that have multiple meanings and social significance. The word *overweight* implies that there is a proper weight and the person has exceeded it. *Obese* is a neutral medical word that simply refers to a physical characteristic, but it has become associated with a long list of negative and pathological implications. *Fat* is a chemical compound made up of carbon, hydrogen, and oxygen, but it also has become associated with negative, judgmental values. Most people are uncomfortable with these words. There is no widely used term for large people that is positive. Because the word *fat* is frequently used in a way that is shaming and punitive, its deliberate use can represent the political reclaiming of a term that is almost universally regarded as negative. Hopefully, this can defuse its potential for damage, and some activists use it to signify a political identity.[5] Reclaiming *fat* as an impartial descriptive term neutralizes its power to injure, which is why I will be using the word throughout this book. If the F-word bothers you, consider what you can do to neutralize it in your own mind.

Binge eating or *overeating* refers to specific behaviors that are also defined differently by different sources. The APA refers to binge eating disorder as "eating in a discrete period of time . . . an amount of food that is definitely larger than what most individuals would eat in a similar period of time under similar circumstances. . . . A sense of lack of control over eating during the episodes."[6] The diagnostic criteria also require a sense of distress, such as guilt, embarrassment, or uncomfortable physical fullness. Although this definition is fairly specific, it is still subjective. An entire large pepperoni pizza might be a binge for a middle-aged women, but it would be a reasonable meal for a college football player. The sense of loss of control is important to the definition of a *binge*, but chronic dieters may experience any relaxing of restraint as loss of control, even if it is not accompanied by increased intake.

There is a difference between characteristics and behaviors. Fat and thin are traits or characteristics, like short and tall. Eating, overeating, restricting, and dieting are behaviors that can be changed. Obesity and overeating are often referred to as if they are interchangeable, when, in reality, they are not even in the same category.

Sometimes anorexia and overeating are referred to as "opposite ends of a spectrum," but, in fact, all the eating disorders are attempts to respond to cultural expectations of thinness. Deb Burgard has suggested that we rename the entire category "disorders of the pursuit of weight loss."[7]

Other terms that are worth considering here are *chronic dieters, restrictive eaters*, and *restrained eaters*. All these refer to people who have been "watching their weight" for periods of time, perhaps most of their lives. Even if someone is not currently on a specific diet but is still focusing on weight loss, that person is eating restrictively. Any attempts to limit intake, whether of calories, fat grams, portion sizes, or certain foods for the purpose of weight loss, is restrictive eating.

Diets Do Not Work

While standing in the checkout line at the local grocery store, it is easy to get a thumbnail sketch of our culture's obsession with weight loss. Almost every magazine cover contains at least one headline exhorting us to "Trim

Down Two Dress Sizes by the Holidays" or "Walk Off Fifteen Pounds" or to try "New Fat-Busting Secrets from the Far East" as well as "Fifteen Fabulous Low-Carb Chocolate Desserts." Why is this?

It is because headlines like that sell magazines—that's why! The dieting industry in this country is a $64 billion a year industry.[8] That means that a whole lot of people are making a whole lot of money by convincing all of us that we are too fat and that we can lose weight if we just buy their product, their program, their food, their book, their video, or their equipment. Those companies advertise in magazines that promote the kind of thinking they want, with articles that keep us grasping for the elusive secret answer that will finally make us thin. Unfortunately, of course, the secret does not exist. However, if everyone knew that, the weight loss industry would not be able to make such a fortune.

The (alleged) "Obesity Epidemic" seems to get more and more press coverage as time goes by, but there are more questions than answers. It is certainly true that people are heavier, on average, than they were 20 or 50 years ago, but there is no one simple explanation for it. A few of the many factors that contribute to it include the following:

- People are living longer, and older people tend to be heavier.
- Most occupations today require significantly less physical activity than in the past.
- Food is more available due to efficient agricultural, storage, and transportation technology.
- Leisure activities are increasingly sedentary.
- Marketing research has shown that there is more money to be made selling appealing, high-fat, high-sodium, ready-to-eat food than more nutritionally dense food, which is time consuming to prepare.
- Fewer people smoke cigarettes.
- Dieting teaches your body to be fatter on less food.

Let me repeat that last one: dieting teaches your body to be fatter on less food. A major contributor to the obesity epidemic that is overlooked or actively ignored is the presumed treatment: dieting. Research, and many individuals' personal experiences, shows that dieting, in the long run, teaches the body to be fatter on less food. This is where the yo-yo pattern originates. A person starts what appears to be a reasonable diet, loses a few pounds, stops losing, gets discouraged, resumes eating what she wants, and gains back all the lost weight, plus a little more. There is a very reasonable explanation for this.

Consider our cave dweller ancestors 50,000 years ago. Food was sometimes plentiful but usually scarce. Much of the focus of survival involved trying to find enough food and somehow store it for times of scarcity.

A person whose body was able to store energy in the form of fat was more likely to survive to reproduce and pass on that characteristic. In the event of a famine, drought, or a long winter, survivors were those whose metabolisms could slow down enough to maintain life on a severely reduced intake. As soon as the next harvest time arrived, those individuals would eat their fill, and their lower metabolisms would enable them to regain all the lost weight, plus add a few more pounds as insurance against the next time of scarcity. The skinny ones died.

Human genetic characteristics have changed very little since then, but our access to food has changed dramatically, and fairly recently, from an historical perspective. Consider the Pilgrims. During the first winter in the New World, many of them died of malnutrition and the related increased susceptibility to disease. The reason that the first Thanksgiving involved such a huge amount and variety of food was not just because they had all been hungry for a long time. It was also because most of that food could not be saved or preserved and would not be available for another year; they needed to eat it while they could. In this day and age, anyone with money or food stamps and access to a grocery store can have turkey, vegetables, and pumpkin pie any day of the year. As long as we can pay for it, it is available.

Physically, the human body reacts to a diet in the same way that our ancestors reacted to a famine. A reduction in energy intake causes a drop in metabolism. The longer the deprivation lasts, the more efficient the body becomes at maintaining itself with less fuel. At the same time, decreased nutrition causes the person to become hyper-vigilant regarding food. In other words, the person notices every food cue in the environment, much like a starved animal will seek out any minimal sign of something edible, while a well-fed animal will walk by without noticing. The dieting individual is distracted by every restaurant, grocery store, and fast-food outlet between home and work and salivates in response to food commercials on television. An adequately nourished person thinks about food only when hungry or at mealtime.

In any living organism, there is a strong physiological drive to eat to obtain energy. The longer it is denied, the stronger it gets. It can be compared to the physiological drive to sleep. The classic example is of the college student who has slept only two hours a night for a week while studying for finals. Then he gets in his car after his last test to drive home for break. Once on the highway, his eyelids droop, and his head nods. We all know what he is supposed to do. We all know that the only wise course is to pull over and take a nap, because we all know that he cannot stay awake simply by an act of "willpower." Yet, when the dieter finally succumbs to the overwhelming physical drive to eat, she will generally berate herself (and be berated by those around her) as not having enough "willpower."

In addition to the physical aspects of hunger, human beings also experience the psychological complications of deprivation. Dieters are typically required to give up or severely limit their favorites foods. The more deprived they feel, the harder it is to maintain that elusive "willpower." Consequently, sooner or later, they abandon their diet.

Hunger causes the dieter to eat more, and deprivation influences her choices. Her metabolism is operating at high efficiency to maintain her weight on the previously low intake. Now her body—like those of the Pilgrims and cave dwellers before her—uses the extra intake to replace the lost pounds and pack on a few extra to prepare for the next famine.

Dieting teaches your body to be fatter on less food.

Repeated dieting teaches your body to binge eat.

Setpoint

The dieting industry can only operate if people accept the premise that weight is mutable, something that can be changed with enough effort. In fact, there is a considerable body of information that supports the concept of the *setpoint*, which is the idea that weight is mostly controlled by genetics and that we are each programmed to maintain a weight within a certain, relatively small range, which is extremely difficult to change. Many of us are genetically programmed to change weight at certain ages or in response to certain conditions. The purpose of dieting is to force the body to weigh less than the setpoint. Many people are able to lose weight, but the vast majority regain it because the body vigorously defends the setpoint.

The line between what we think we can control and what we cannot control has been deliberately blurred. There is a difference between behavior and characteristics. Eating, dieting, and exercise are all behaviors, and we make choices about them. Height, eye color, bone structure, visual acuity, and many other physical characteristics are not things we can make choices about. Weight and body composition are, to a large extent, physical characteristics over which we have very little control. However, there is a great deal of money being made because we have been taught to *believe* we can change weight permanently if we just keep searching for the right program.

It would seem obvious that the high failure rate is because diets do not work. In addition, the activity of dieting is not simply useless; it is harmful. Repeated "failures" at dieting erode self-esteem and undermine trust in one's own judgment, resulting in guilt, disgust, self-recrimination, and self-loathing. "Failed" dieting can worsen physical measures such as blood pressure, insulin resistance, and cholesterol levels. Weight cycling is dangerous to physical and mental well-being.

In both research and in medical treatment, the concept of *informed consent* is a very important ethical consideration. People deserve to know all of the possible benefits and risks before agreeing to treatment or to participating in a research project. This is why television and print advertisements for medications have a long list of possible side effects and why you have to sign a release before having a simple procedure in your doctor's office: legally, you must be informed of everything that could possibly go wrong, and you have the right to change your mind if you do not like the risks. You have the right to be fully informed and to make your own decision.

The dieting industry has managed to avoid complying with this expectation, aside from the tiny "results not typical" statement at the bottom of some advertisements. They would not make much money if they had to state, "You have a 95 percent chance of regaining the weight you lose, and maybe more, while possibly harming your health in the process."

"But Being Fat Is So Unhealthy!"

In truth, you cannot tell anything about a person's health or behavior by looking at his or her weight. In the next chapter, we will look at the evidence demonstrating that attempts to lose weight do not work and that there is a difference between weight and health. Then, we will address what actually does work to improve physical, emotional, and social health, based on the Health At Every Size principles.

The Underpants Rule

The incomparable Ragen Chastain originated the Underpants Rule, which I will refer to from time to time (see figure 1.1).

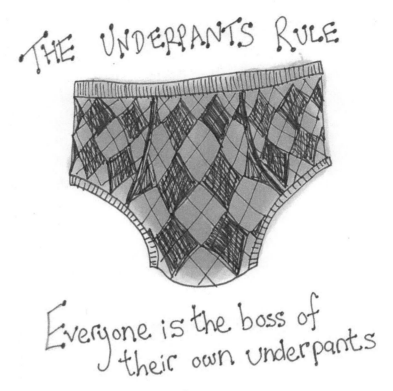

THE UNDERPANTS RULE

Everyone is the boss of their own underpants

You get to make choices about your life.

Other people get to make choices about their lives.

Our choices aren't other people's business unless we ask.

Other people's choices aren't our business unless they ask.

Figure 1.1 (Words: Ragen Chastain, www.danceswithfat.org. Image: Pesky Chloe, www.lifesbigcanvas.co.uk.)

CHAPTER TWO

The Science of Weight and Health

"Everybody Knows . . ."

Once upon a time, everyone knew that the world was flat, that fog caused malaria, and that drinking enough milk cured ulcers. We now know that the world is round, that malaria is caused by a microorganism spread by mosquitoes, and that ulcers are best treated with antibiotics. Meanwhile, the amount of commonly believed misinformation about weight and health remains widespread and damaging. This misinformation can, for the most part, be summed up in three myths:

1. Body weight is under an individual's control.
2. Eating more calories than the body needs causes weight gain, and eating less causes sustainable weight loss (also known as "calories in, calories out").
3. Weight is a measure of health.
   a. Weight loss improves health, and weight gain harms health.
   b. Thinner people are healthier that heavier people.

A considerable amount of science and research literature disproves these assumptions, but before we get to that, it may be helpful to say a few things about how to evaluate information.

Background: How Research Works

A couple of years ago, I found myself in a conversation with a woman who was going on and on about a supplement that she was selling that purportedly caused weight loss. I was trying to be polite, but I finally asked her, "Do you have any peer-reviewed journal articles that support your claim?"

She looked at me blankly and then smiled. "Oh, you mean testimonials! Yes, we have lots of those!"

This incident illustrated for me that people who do not have careers in science, medicine, research, or academia may be unaware of the many variables involved in evaluating information. I have attempted to explain some of these variables in, hopefully, a nonboring way. (If you do have a career in science, medicine, research, academia, or something related, feel free to skip ahead to the next section.)

Peer review is a process in which qualified professionals in the relevant field anonymously review a submission for publication. It is a way to ensure the quality and accuracy of information in professional journals. It includes fact-checking as well as assessment of the validity of the research methods, data collection, evaluation, and conclusions. Until the reviewers are satisfied, the paper will not be published in a professional journal. In contrast, articles published in general magazines and newspapers, in print or online, may have been reviewed by an editor for grammar and writing style and may or may not have had the information checked for accuracy, depending on the standards of the publication.

Testimonials are personal statements about a product or program and usually fall in the category of advertising. The people making the statements may or may not have a financial interest in the product being promoted. Testimonials also rarely include a time frame; "This worked for me!" may be about something that has only worked for a week or two. These statements can also be word of mouth, or what I think of as "my next-door neighbor's babysitter's niece" stories, as in "My next-door neighbor's babysitter's niece (or my hairdresser's boyfriend's daughter, etc.) tried this product/treatment/supplement for her asthma/headache/ingrown toenail, and it worked for her!"

Testimonials are fine if you are deciding which book to purchase at the airport bookstore. But if you are considering treatment for a health issue, don't you want more reliable information? For instance, to be approved by the FDA, medications must go through a rigorous set of tests to show that they are safe and effective. This involves, among other things, a *controlled, double-blind study*. This means that half of the participants are given the medication, and the other half are given a placebo, which has no effect. The participants do not know which one they are taking and neither do the researchers who are evaluating the effectiveness—thus the term *double blind*.

This makes sense because the researchers can subtly influence the outcome if they know who is taking the placebo and who is taking the real thing. If the medication being studied were, for instance, a sleep aid, the researcher probably would not ask, "Your sleep has improved, hasn't it?" or

"Your sleep isn't any better, is it?" But even if the questions are strictly controlled, the tone of voice and a lift of eyebrows can encourage a certain response. This is why the researchers evaluating the outcome are kept "blind" as to who gets the pill and who gets the placebo. (Researchers have researched this question at great length and have found any number of subtle ways that the people gathering the information can influence outcomes. Simply being observed can change participants' behavior.)

Unfortunately, approaches to weight loss are rarely, if ever, subjected to the same rigorous evaluation. Many products are marketed that claim to change the body with little or no evidence beyond testimonials. They may even use the term "scientifically proven" in the marketing materials but become evasive if anyone asks to see the science. I once encountered a salesperson at a bridal show who was selling a "wrap" that claimed to contain herbs that would somehow reduce the size of "problem" body areas, such as the abdomen, thighs, or arms. She was selling the system to entire bridal parties so they could all be "more slender" on the wedding day. I asked about the evidence that it worked, and she referred me to the website, which contained nothing but more marketing hype. A double-blind study for this product might compare her wraps with other wraps that did not contain the active ingredient (but smelled the same) and have measurements taken by someone who did not know who had used which product, as measuring tapes are notoriously inaccurate, depending on how snugly they are pulled.

This brings up another concern: how accurate is the measurement? In research terminology, this is referred to as *reliability*. Will the measurement be the same when taken by different people or in different circumstances? A good example is height. A measurement of your adult height (in bare feet) should be the same at home or in a doctor's office, today or next month. In contrast, blood pressure can be tricky to measure because it changes in response to circumstances, such as having the doctor walk into the room (this is known as *white coat hypertension*). Several measures of blood pressure may be necessary to identify a trend or average because a single measurement is not always reliable.

If a measure is *reliable* from one circumstance to another, that does not necessarily mean that it is *valid*. The term *validity* refers to how good the measure is at actually measuring what is being evaluated. For instance, taking your temperature is not a valid measurement of depression, even if your temperature is reliable from one day to the next. Similarly, body weight is not a valid measure of health, even if it is reliable.

In general conversation, the word *significant* means important or meaningful, as in, "That was a significant event in my life." In research, one way the word *significant* is used is to assess how sure we are that it did not happen by accident or coincidence. (I am simplifying somewhat.) This is also referred to as *probability* and is usually represented in research literature as "*p* =." A *p* value of 0.05 means, "We are 95 percent certain that this did not happen by accident or coincidence." A p value of 0.01 means 99 percent certainty, and $p = 0.001$ is 99.9 percent certainty. Statisticians, who are very clever, have numerous equations for determining these values under different circumstances. Something can have statistical significance and still not be relevant. An example of how this might be seen in weight loss literature is a study where a number of people are put on weight loss diets, and half of them are also given a medication. They all lose weight, but the participants who took the medication have "significantly more" weight loss. However, the details of the study might reveal that the participants without the medication lost an average of 4 pounds and those with the medication lost an average of 6 pounds. That difference may not be meaningful to the participants, but the evaluation of the data shows that it is statistically likely that the difference is because of the medication; therefore, it is statistically significant.

The word *theory* is used in everyday conversation to refer to ideas or guesses. Researchers make a clear distinction between a *theory* and a *hypothesis*. A well-designed research project usually has one specific question that it studies. Using the above example, the researchers would specify an *experimental hypothesis*, "Use of this medication will result in increased weight loss," and a *null hypothesis*, "Use of this medication will make no difference in weight loss." To support the hypothesis, they want to show a 95 percent likelihood that the null hypothesis is wrong. This sounds complicated, and it is, but the nitty-gritty details of research are easier to sort out using this terminology. An idea or hypothesis is only considered a theory after a considerable amount of evidence has been collected to support it. A theory is something that explains observable fact, such as gravity, that is difficult to definitively prove or disprove. When someone says, "That's just a theory," they probably do not understand how the word is being used.

An additional concept that is important in understanding research literature is the difference between *correlation* and *causation*. Two things can happen together, but that does not mean one caused the other. If you wash your car and it rains, did the activity of washing the car cause it to rain? If it only happened once, is that a coincidence? How many times would you have to wash the car and have it rain, or not wash the car and have it not rain, before you could say that the correlation is statistically significant? Even if the correlation is statistically significant, that does not prove that one caused the other. For instance, the murder rate is highest in the month of August; there is also more ice cream consumed in August than any other month in the year. Does that mean that eating ice cream causes murder? Or does committing murder cause people to eat more ice cream? Or perhaps the high temperatures in August cause some people to become so irritable that they are not safe to be around and cause other people to eat more ice cream.

Another related problem with the evaluation of information is *interpretation*. Often, a legitimate, well-done piece of research is published in a reputable journal, and a press release is distributed. A reporter, whose job it is to sell newspapers, picks up one piece of information from the press release, out of context, and writes an eye-grabbing headline. Readers accept that interpretation as true without knowing what else was involved or what the researchers actually found.

Research about Weight Loss

The weight loss industry is big business in the United States, generating about $60 billion a year.[1] The people making that money need us to believe that losing weight is necessary and also possible if we buy whatever it is that they are selling. It is all a lie; no approach works long term for more than a tiny fraction of people who try it. However, those same people who profit from selling this idea have considerable influence over what we see in magazines and newspapers and on television. They are even able to influence what medical professionals think about weight and health. They stand to lose money if the truth about their approaches becomes widely known.

The actual scientific information about weight and health is very complicated, and there is still much that we do not know. Even studies published in peer-reviewed journals may have flaws because of the generally accepted assumption that weight loss is always good and always possible. Studies that report "successful" weight loss approaches usually have several things in common. Frequently, the study follows participants for 3 or 4 months, perhaps as long as a year, but rarely longer than that. These short-term results are then used to inaccurately predict long-term effects. Often, the maximum weight loss was achieved after 3 or 4 months, and weight regain has started by month 12. The weight at the one-year mark is still considered a success because it is lower than the starting weight; however the continued weight gain after one year is not addressed. In addition, people often drop out of weight loss research studies because they cannot follow the regime without great distress, they feel like a failure, or they are not losing as fast as they think they should. If "success" is only reported for those individuals who are still participating at the end, we do not know about the others, who may account for half or more of those who started. Sometimes follow-up weight is self-reported rather than measured and may not be reliable. (How many people do you suppose have a driver's license that accurately reports their weight?)

Another question concerns how *success* is defined. Many studies consider a loss of 3–5 percent of the beginning body weight to be a success. This means that a person who weighs 300 pounds would be successful when losing 15 pounds. At 285, that person is probably still going to be lectured by friends and family about weight loss. Rarely will a 5 percent weight loss move a person from one body mass index (BMI) category to another. A person with a BMI over 30 is unlikely to maintain a weight loss of even 5 percent and is extremely unlikely to achieve a weight in the "normal" category.[2]

Sometimes researchers use weight or BMI as an indication of nutrition and physical activity, primarily because it is so easy to measure. Accurately measuring nutritional intake and amounts of exercise is very challenging, but using weight as a proxy is not valid, as previously discussed. Many people with high BMIs eat a lot of fruits and vegetables and are physically active, while many skinny folks eat mostly processed food and are sedentary. Yet, the myths about weight are so unquestioned that research is still published that uses BMI as a proxy measure for nutrition and physical activity.

While we are on the subject, individual BMI is a notoriously flawed measure of health. It is simply a ratio of weight to height. The BMI was developed in the early days of the field of statistics by a Belgian mathematician named Quetelet and was then called the Quetelet index. It was designed to measure large groups of people; it was not meant to be used to evaluate individuals. It does not account for body composition, such as muscle mass or height, which results in athletes and tall people having higher BMIs. When it first began to be used to evaluate individuals, which happened fairly recently, a BMI of 20–27 was considered "normal," 28–32 was "overweight," and above 32 was "obese." In 1998, under pressure from the diet industry, the World Health Organization changed the standards to 20–25 as "normal," 26–30 as "overweight," and above 30 as "obese." As Linda Bacon says in her excellent book *Health at Every Size*, "Thanks to this task force, one magical night in June of 1998 some 29 million Americans went to bed with average figures and woke up fat."[3]

At some point, "normal" expanded to 18.5–25. When I worked on an inpatient eating disorder treatment program from 1985 to 1993, we did not talk about BMI. We used a formula, accepted by health insurers, to estimate the "ideal body weight" for adolescent/young adult women. The diagnostic criteria threshold required for a diagnosis of anorexia nervosa was below 85 percent. A BMI of 18.5 percent meets that criteria but is now considered "normal."

When you see a headline about the increase in the number of people who are overweight or obese in the last 30 years, which criteria are they using? Comparing numbers from 1995 to 2015 may be comparing two different measures. Are Americans really getting heavier or did the criteria change?

The widely used term *obesity epidemic* is designed to strike fear in our hearts, but the average weight of Americans has only increased by 12–15 pounds in the last 30 years.[4] Some of this change is likely related to the fact that people are living longer, and older people tend to be heavier. Characterizing weight gain as an epidemic disease has been largely driven by financial interests. The idea that obesity is deadly justifies promoting drugs and surgeries with dangerous side effects and expecting them to be covered by health insurance.[5]

What Science Tells Us about Weight, Health, and Weight Loss

There is an enormous and growing body of literature debunking the myths about weight and health.[6] It is beyond the scope of this chapter to review more than a small portion of it, so I have tried to provide a helpful overview.

The concept of the *set point* was introduced in 1982 by William Bennett and Joel Gurin in their excellent (and, sadly, now out of print) book *The Dieter's Dilemma*.[7] The theory has been widely debated since then and has a growing body of evidence to support it. The *set point* refers to a weight range that is different for each person and that is defended by numerous physiological mechanisms. This allows the body to adapt to varying availability of food and activity. Adults who make no conscious effort to change their weight usually maintain a stable weight over time. The set point for weight is primarily determined by genetics, but it can also be influenced by medication, environmental chemicals, stress, illness, microbiota in the gut, and several other factors that are only now being studied.

A fascinating study was published in 1986 examining the genetic influences on weight. Five hundred and forty Danish adults adopted as infants were compared to their biological and adoptive parents in terms of weight. The researchers found a very strong and significant correlation with biological parents and none at all with adoptive parents.[8] In other words, the baby of two fat parents grew up to be fat even if the adoptive parents were thin, and vice versa. Food and eating patterns in the household had minimal influence.

There is strong evidence that dieting for weight loss causes the set point to increase. The body has many ways to defend the set point; when weight drops below the natural range, the metabolism slows down, and hunger increases. Muscle tissue is lost with lost weight but regained as fat tissue, which also contributes to a slower metabolism. Conversely, people who voluntarily overeat have been shown to have increased metabolism and decreased hunger.[9]

Defining *dieting* as a voluntary, self-imposed famine, Macpherson-Sánchez[10] makes a compelling argument that dieting—supported by public policy, the medical community, and the $60 billion per year weight loss industry—is a major cause of the "obesity epidemic." Additionally, focus on the undesirability of heavier weight is linked to weight stigma in the culture and internalized body dissatisfaction in people of all sizes.

Available information has told us for decades that deliberate attempts to lose weight almost always fail.[11-22] Many people can lose weight over a period of a few months, but they then begin to regain it, even if they continue to fol-low the same behaviors that initially resulted in loss. In most studies, some weight is regained by the end of the first year, with regain continuing until body weight is higher than at the beginning of the attempt to lose. Many stud-ies only follow people for a few months; those that follow participants longer find that most weight is regained by year three. Perhaps 5 percent of dieters are able to maintain a partial weight loss by year five, and most of them spend an extraordinary amount of time focusing on maintaining it, essentially behaving in a way that is consistent with a diagnosis of anorexia nervosa.[23–28]

As long ago as 1959, Stunkard and McLaren-Hume documented the per-vasive lack of success in weight loss treatment programs and pointed out that doctors often dismissed patients who failed to lose weight as "uncooperative" and "gluttonous."[29] They also stated that weight loss treatments were poten-tially dangerous and should not be undertaken lightly, if at all. In 1982, Wooley and Wooley expressed concerns that eating disordered behavior was being touted as a weight loss approach despite evidence that thin people were not healthier than heavy people, that weight is more complicated than energy balance, and that the prevailing belief was that thinness is worth any price, including health.[30]

Research from 1995 and earlier documented that the human body will adapt metabolically to maintain weight when intake is restricted in an attempt to lose weight.[31,32] Research continues to support the concept that the human body responds with biological adaptations to maintain weight in response to restricted intake.[33] As energy intake falls, hunger increases, mak-ing sustained weight loss all but impossible.[34–36]

"But being fat is so unhealthy!" As often as this statement is repeated, it is not supported by the evidence. The assumption that body fat causes health problems is not well supported by the data.[37] Weight and BMI are both highly inaccurate measures of health.[38] A more accurate evaluation of health involves measuring cardiometabolic abnormalities, including blood pressure, choles-terol levels, insulin resistance, and C-reactive protein (a measure of inflam-mation). One large study found that nearly a third of people with a "normal" weight had metabolic abnormalities, while half of "overweight" people and nearly a third of "obese" adults were metabolically healthy.[39] Even in people who have some cardiometabolic abnormalities, it is difficult to sort out the impact of weight versus the effect of social stigma.[40]

In other words, thin people are sometimes unhealthy, fat people are some-times healthy, and weight stigma probably contributes to the poor health outcomes that are commonly associated with being fat. Internal and external stigma cause chronic stress, which is associated with heart disease, hyper-tension, hypercholesterolemia, and diabetes, and the amount of discrepancy between actual and ideal body weight is more predictive of health problems than BMI.[41] In other words, being unhappy about one's weight may be worse for your health than the actual weight.

A study from the Centers for Disease Control and Prevention found that, categorizing people with the standard BMI measure, those in the "over-weight" BMI category had lower mortality than those who were a "normal" weight, and those in the level considered "grade one obesity (BMI 30–35)" did not have higher mortality than those considered "normal."[42] Thin people do not necessarily live longer than fat people. Research literature continues to expand to include studies involving the "obesity paradox," in which heavier people have better outcomes than thinner peers when faced with many diseases, surgeries, or injuries.

There are a number of health conditions that seen to correlate with higher weight, but that does not prove causation. Just like the earlier example of ice cream consumption and murder in August, both may be caused by a third variable. For instance, insulin resistance appears to cause both diabetes and weight gain. The insulin resistance happens first. Unfortunately, the prevailing belief that being heavy *causes* diabetes results in many people feeling unnecessarily guilty about creating their own illness, which interferes with their ability to take good care of themselves.

Even if higher weight might be related to poorer health, there is little reason to think that reducing weight will result in improved health measures. Bombak's comprehensive review of weight loss interventions documents their failure to improve health.[43] Meanwhile, individuals are encouraged to engage in disordered eating behaviors and are praised when they do so. Pursuit of weight loss is not simply a waste of time; it results in negative outcomes in terms of physical, mental, and social health. Health promotion programs that focus on weight loss have been shown to result in body dissatisfaction, discrimination, eating disorders, and even death.[44] Restrictive eating in weight loss efforts is associated with cognitive impairment, such as difficulty concentrating and thinking clearly.[45] Tomiyama et al. found that dieting is correlated with increased stress and cortisol levels, which are linked to several negative health outcomes, including heart disease, impaired immune function, cancer, diabetes, and, ironically, weight gain.[46] Even people who are at a "normal" weight and are eating restrictively to avoid being "overweight" are more likely to gain weight in response to the restriction.[47] In both thin and heavy people, unhappiness about weight, rather than the weight itself, is associated with increased likelihood of illness.[48–50] Psychological distress and body dissatisfaction are associated with poorer health and health behaviors and higher metabolic abnormalities.[51–56]

Weight cycling is the term used to describe deliberate weight loss followed by regain, also known as *yo-yo dieting*. This process is iatrogenic, in that it causes health problems in and of itself. Many of the problems blamed on high weight may, in fact, be caused by weight cycling. Variability in weight is associated with increased cardiovascular disease, diabetes, and early death.[57]

The general belief that weight loss always results in improved health is not supported by the research. In a study that reviewed 21 well-designed trials of weight loss that had at least a two-year follow-up, no clear relationship was found between weight loss and health.[58] Studies that compare the health of thin people to heavy people cannot conclude that weight loss improves health. To do that, we would need to compare thin people to previously heavy people who have become thin, and we do not have a sample of people who have maintained weight loss to make that comparison. "The entire prescription of weight loss assumes that if heavier people lose weight they will have the same risks as a never-been-heavier person, but that has never been tested. The data are silent on the premise that a weight-suppressed person will have the same health risks as a never-been-heavier person."[59]

Understanding the relationship between weight and health is further complicated by weight bias in the medical field. When medical professionals focus on weight as a problem, it distracts from other concerns. Quality of care is affected. When patients experience negative attitudes and disrespectful treatment because of their size, they are less likely to seek treatment when appropriate.[60–64] Larger women have been shown to delay cancer screenings because of negative experiences with providers, and they are more likely to avoid care if they have had more failed weight loss attempts.[65] It is impossible to fully evaluate the effect of weight on health when stigma is a barrier to accessing health care.

Meanwhile, the nearly certain inability to maintain weight loss is associated with decreased self-esteem and increased symptoms of depression.[66] As an alternative, weight-neutral interventions focus on improving health-related behaviors, such as exercise, eating a wider variety of foods, and size acceptance. A review that compared weight loss approaches with weight-neutral approaches found that weight-neutral approaches resulted in better psychological and physiological outcomes as well as better participant retention. The authors questioned the ethical aspects of recommending weight loss interventions when they are associated with poorer health outcomes and increased psychological distress.[67] A focus on increased physical activity instead of reduced weight is increasingly seen as beneficial.[68]

Several behaviors have been shown to improve health independent of weight. A study that followed almost 12,000 people for an average of 14 years compared mortality hazard ratio and number of healthy habits. The four behaviors measured were avoiding tobacco use, moderating alcohol intake, engaging in regular exercise, and eating at least five fruits and vegetables daily. Participants were categorized by BMI into "normal," "overweight," and "obese." Engaging in more healthy behaviors correlated with lower mortality across weight categories, with people in the "obese" category showing the most benefit.[69]

Another study that compared weight-normative (focused on weight loss) to weight-inclusive (focused on behaviors) approaches found that a focus on weight was associated with adverse physical and psychological outcomes as well as increased blame, shame, and stigma with decreased well-being; that dieting was linked to preventable barriers to health; that weight stigma was associated with increased intake; and that a focus on the weight-normative approach became a self-perpetuating dogma. Weight-inclusive programs, on the other hand, resulted in improvement in health behaviors as well as better physical and psychological measures because people are more likely to engage in good self-care when they feel positively toward their bodies. The authors went on to say that public health messages to "maintain a healthy weight" are unfair and uninformed.[70]

An often overlooked source of information about the body's response to dieting is the starvation experiment that was done during World War II.[71] Officials in the U.S. government were aware that many people in Europe were at risk of starvation because of the disruptions to food production as a result of the war. They assigned Ancel Keys, "the government's dietician," to gather information about ways to refeed people after starvation. Keys (more popularly known as the inventor of the K-ration) gathered 36 conscientious objectors who volunteered to participate in a study of starvation as an alternative to military service. It became the only known controlled study of human starvation, and it is likely the only one there ever will be because no research board would approve it now. It was brutal!

Initially, the young, healthy men were fed a normal amount—about 3,500 calories a day—while extensive medical tests documented everything that the researchers knew how to document. After three months, the men were cut back to half rations, 1,550 calories a day, for six months. They were required to participate in considerable physical activity while their metabolisms were rigorously measured. Their weight dropped rapidly, and their metabolic rates slowed within a few days of the decreased intake. They became irritable, depressed, lethargic, and introverted. Some experienced severe mood swings. They developed intense preoccupation with food, taking hours to eat a meal and using large amounts of seasoning. Some of them spent their free time reading cookbooks, planning menus, and making grocery lists. They thought about food all the time and found it difficult to concentrate on anything else. They avoided activities such as work or study, even recreation. They lost interest in sex. They neglected personal grooming, and they became physically weaker. They were unable to follow the honor system of staying on the diet, sometimes finding access to food, bingeing, and then engaging in tearful self-recrimination. Access to coffee, tea, and chewing gum had to be limited when the men used excessive amounts to distract themselves from hunger.

The refeeding period of the experiment involved different levels of intake for different participants; however, they all reported insatiable hunger. Even the men who were eating 4,000 calories a day reported being unsatisfied. At the final banquet, when they were allowed to eat without restriction, many of them became ill from overeating. Even when gorging to the point of physical discomfort, they remained hungry. It took several months of restored intake and restored weight before their attitudes about food began to return to normal. Some of them never completely regained their ability to feel satisfied.

The study established the association of weight suppression and restricted intake with psychological and physical complications. Dr. Keys was not interested in eating disorders, but his meticulous notes have provided information for researchers and clinicians since the publication of *The Biology of Human Starvation* in 1950. It consists of two volumes of over 800 pages each, which is not light reading. If you are interested in learning more about this fascinating study, I recommend Todd Tucker's 2006 book *The Great Starvation Experiment: The Heroic Men Who Starved So That Millions Could Live*.[72] This study could not be repeated today because of the numerous ethical concerns, yet diets that restrict intake even more severely are routinely recommended for those who are encouraged to lose weight!

A couple of decades later, another researcher, Ethan Sims, wanted to see what would happen if he could make thin people temporarily fat.[73] He started with university students (remember, this was before weight stigma made people terrified of gaining weight) who deliberately overate to try to gain. They found it nearly impossible to increase their weight by even a small amount. He tried again with a more sedentary group, prisoners (again, this was before approval was required from ethics boards). He chose lean men who did not have a family history of obesity. For over six months, the men ate valiantly but struggled to gain. Once they did gain 20 percent above their starting weights, they had to consume about 2,000 *extra* calories a day to maintain it. They found the experience very unpleasant. After the experiment ended, they readily lost the extra weight simply by going back to the way they had eaten before. "If we lived in a world that prized being fat instead of thin, Sims's results might be attributed to the prisoners' lack of character. . . . The difficulties and even failures both groups experienced are some indication of the irrelevance of character to fatness."[74]

A study done in the early 1950s demonstrated the ability of the appetite to adapt to changing energy needs. A cohort of military cadets, whose daily activity level was determined as a group, had their intake and energy expenditures carefully monitored for two weeks. Though they were not consciously managing either one, they ate exactly what they needed for their activity levels. They also demonstrated a two-day lag; they did not eat more on days when they were more active but did eat more two days later.[75] In other words, their bodies did an exquisitely efficient job of balancing energy intake with output, with no conscious effort on their part.

A more recent interesting example is the reality television program *The Biggest Loser*, which was widely watched during its run from 2005 to 2016. Most viewers seemed to believe that the show offered a way for very fat people to become healthier and that the way it portrayed the participants was sympathetic and caring. In fact, it was problematic on many levels. Watching the show was documented to increase anti-fat bias and reinforce the belief that weight is under an individual's control.[76,77] Adolescents who viewed clips expressed more fear of weight gain.[78] The way the participants were treated on the show reinforced the idea that shame and humiliation are useful and reasonable to motivate people to work harder at weight loss, which justifies bullying behavior because "It's for your own good." In the end, it was like any other weight loss attempt, ending in regained weight and slower metabolism.[79] Participants were required to sign nondisclosure agreements, but some have spoken publicly about the physically dangerous workout requirements, the damage and injuries that resulted, and the way the show was edited to misrepresent the reality and make for better entertainment.[80] Meanwhile, the show, and its related products and resorts, became a multimillion-dollar brand.

What a Shame!

Acceptance of the myths that weight is under an individual's control and that weight loss leads to improved health gives rise to the idea that shaming people will motivate them to lose weight. Weight shaming is commonly seen at the dinner table, in the doctor's office, in public health interventions, in reality television, and in advice columns; it is framed as "for your own good." The unexamined assumption behind weight shaming is the belief that weight is a behavior that is individually controllable instead of a characteristic that is extremely resistant to change. Weight stigma does not motivate people to engage in healthy behaviors and is likely to backfire, resulting in poorer health behaviors and outcomes.[81–85] "If stigmatizing fat people worked, it would have done so by now."[86] Meanwhile, a substantial body of research supports the idea that size and body acceptance correlates with improved health and improved health behaviors.[87–94]

Weight stigma leads to body dissatisfaction and distress, which has implications for society as well as for individuals. The fact that body shame is common does not make it any less damaging. Body shame and weight stigma reinforce each other, perpetuating a vicious cycle that impairs quality of life in ways that should not be accepted, but are. We will return to an examination of stigma in more detail in chapters 6 and 7.

When all of this information is taken into account, it becomes clear that attempts at weight loss do not work; they make things worse. Interventions that focus on improving behaviors without trying to change body size are more likely to have a good outcome. If we could stop weight stigma and shaming, that would be even better! Accepting and loving one's body as it is right now leads to improved health behaviors that have a much better chance of leading to improved health.

What about Food Addicts?

The concept of food addiction seems to be appealing to many people, but the evidence is sketchy at best.[95-98] The elimination of an entire food category certainly can make decisions easier in the short term, but it is not helpful long term.

Part of the difficulty is in how we define *addiction*. Addictive substances are not needed in the body until they are introduced, when the presence of the substance creates the need. The original definition of an *addictive substance* includes needing an increasing dose to achieve the effect desired and physiologic withdrawal symptoms when it is not available. By this definition, alcohol, caffeine, nicotine, heroin, and benzodiazepines, among others, are addictive. For instance, I am addicted to caffeine; if I do not get my morning cup of coffee, I develop a pounding headache, which is unpleasant but survivable. In contrast, withdrawal for alcohol is potentially fatal, which is the reason for inpatient detox treatment for people addicted to alcohol. Many medications that are used to treat a symptom are not addictive, but the symptom will return when the medication is discontinued. For example, antihistamines are not addictive, but missing a dose usually results in a return of the symptom of sneezing, which is not the same as withdrawal.

Human beings are born needing food and water. We do not become addicted by consuming them; we will die without them. Food cravings and uncontrollable bingeing are related to restriction, which we will address in more detail in chapter 3.

The 12-step model for addiction treatment, also known as the abstinence model, is the predominant and accepted approach in the United States for treatment of substance abuse. Many people with substance abuse problems have benefited from the abstinence model of treatment, which includes, among other things, an intention to abstain, to never use the substance again. It would be convenient if we could apply that model to eating, but it does not work. How do you define *abstinence*? We all need to eat several times a day, every day. It is possible to abstain from alcohol, or caffeine, or nicotine forever. It is not possible to abstain from food.

Abstinence requires identifying something specific as the problem. Treatment approaches for weight concerns that are based on the concept of food addiction require that people completely give up sugar, white flour, high-fat foods, or snacks and follow an extensive set of rules—forever. Initially, there is a certain relief in having fewer choices, and the limits imposed usually result in temporary weight loss. Eventually, though, many folks find themselves craving the forbidden food and falling off the wagon, with the attendant guilt and shame. At the same time, some people find a certain amount of comfort in the idea of having an addiction because it implies that they cannot help their behavior.

The argument for food addiction rests, in part, on animal studies that show that eating certain foods, especially sugar, affect the dopamine system in the brain. Drugs of abuse activate the reward circuit, the pleasure center, in the brain, which increases the neurotransmitter dopamine. Consuming highly palatable foods lights up the dopaminergic pathways, but so does laughter, music, or seeing someone you love.[99]

Measurements have been developed to try to identify people with "food addiction" based on the criteria used to define substance abuse, but more people self-identify as food addicted than meet the criteria.[100] In the literature that I have seen regarding research into the concept of "food addiction," there is considerable overlap with binge eating disorder and a focus on weight loss. This reflects, in my opinion, an unexamined bias on the part of the researchers, who do not ask about dieting history. Restrained eaters (also known as chronic dieters) and self-identified food addicts similarly report eating in response to external cues and rules, less confidence in internal signals of hunger or satiety, more dietary restraint, and less self-control around food.[101] Successful treatment for binge eating disorder includes incorporating all foods and learning to eat in response to internal cues while relinquishing a focus on weight loss. Treating highly palatable foods as a substance that must be avoided at all costs may increase the likelihood of bingeing. Besides, who wants to give up their favorite food forever if it is not necessary?

Why Do We Keep Trying the Same Things When They Do Not Work?

Many people in the research, medical, and business fields have made careers and fortunes promoting the idea that weight loss is desirable and possible. Those people have a lot to lose by reconsidering the information that is available. The following quote by Ronald Fisher (a really smart statistician guy) in 1947 makes a valuable point:

> A scientific career is peculiar in some ways. Its raison d'être is the increase of natural knowledge. Occasionally, therefore, an increase of natural knowledge occurs. But this is tactless, and feelings are hurt. For in some small degree it is inevitable that views previously expounded are shown to be either obsolete or false. Most people, I think, can recognize this and take it in good part if what they have been teaching for ten years or so comes to need a little revision; but undoubtedly take it hard, as a blow to their amour proper, or even as an invasion of the territory they have come to think of as exclusively their own, and they must react with the same ferocity as we can see in the robins and chaffinches these spring days when they resent an intrusion into their little territories. I do not think anything can be done about it. It is inherent in the nature of our profession; but a young scientist may be warned and advised that when he has a jewel to offer for the enrichment of mankind some will certainly wish to turn and rend him.[102]

The weight loss industry and the pharmaceutical industry both have a huge financial stake in promoting weight loss. They do this not only by advertising to the public but also by offering biased information to medical professionals.

Alicia Mundy's excellent book *Dispensing with the Truth: The Victims, the Drug Companies, and the Dramatic Story behind the Battle over Fen-Phen* offers a fascinating account of how the manufacturers of diet pills offered continuing education to physicians in which they inflated the risks of obesity to make their dangerous drugs appear safer in comparison.[103] Additionally, much of the research in the obesity field is funded by some segment of the dieting industry.[104,105] The widely held (but unsupported) belief that weight loss is possible and leads to improved health also limits funding and publication possibilities for weight-neutral research if it is not described as "obesity prevention."[106–109]

In 2007, Mann et al. concluded that "the benefits of dieting are simply too small and the potential harms of dieting are too large for it to be recommended as a safe and effective treatment for obesity."[110] Meanwhile, the weight loss industry is raking in about $60 billion a year, and they control what we read.[111] General media publications (such as women's magazines and Sunday inserts) sell advertising by promoting what the weight loss industry wants to see. It looks something like figure 2.1.

To recap, dieting is bad for you, and attempts at weight loss do not work long term. Weight is not an accurate measure of health. Attempts to lose weight do not make us healthier; in fact, they make us sicker and heavier. A lot of people are making a whole lot of money by convincing us that being fat is terrible and that we can all lose weight by spending our hard-earned money on their ineffective products. They control what we read and see in the general media. They suppress any information that contradicts them.

Does that make you angry? It should. What is the alternative? I am glad you asked; read on.

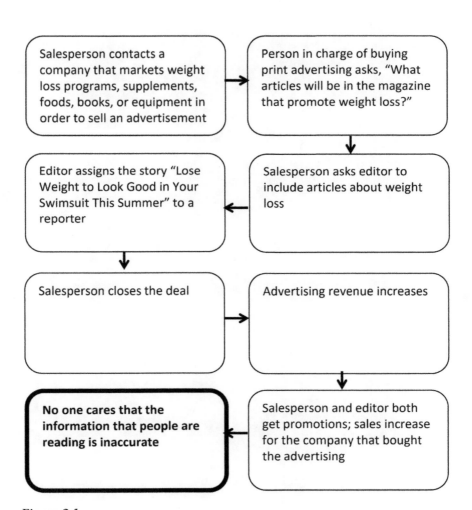

Figure 2.1

CHAPTER THREE

Finding Peace

If you are reading this book, it is probably because you are looking for ways to be at peace with your body and with food. Weight stigma and the relentless social pressure to be thinner have resulted in many, if not most, people in our culture feeling that they are at war with their bodies. The battles in this war take place at the dinner table, at the grocery store, at the gym, and in any place where eating or thinking about eating occurs. How do we heal the damaged relationships with our bodies? How do we heal our damaged relationships with food? The process may not be easy or quick, but it can be done.

One of the unintended consequences of the "war on obesity" is the huge increase in anxiety about eating. Nourishing our bodies should not be a source of fear and distress, but most people have come to accept those feelings as normal. This discomfort affects everyone of all sizes, although in different ways. The experience of the shame and stigma directed at fat people for their natural body size is debilitatingly painful, and it indirectly impacts those around them, as well. People who are naturally slender are terrified of gaining weight and then being treated the same way, so they, too, develop anxiety about everything they put in their mouths. It is important to acknowledge both of these processes as true: fat people have a very difficult time living in our society, and not-fat people are influenced by observing the abuse that fat people endure.

Finding your way back to a positive relationship with your body and eating may be a challenging undertaking. When you get discouraged, it helps to remember what the pursuit of thinness has cost in the past. This might be a good time to make a list of what those costs have been. How much money have you paid for diet programs that did not work? What events have you avoided, or not enjoyed, because of the food that would be served? What delicious meals have you been deprived of? What social interactions have you missed? How has your quality of life been sacrificed on the altar of an unattainable thinner body?

Quality of life cannot be measured on a scale.

Health At Every Size: The Peace Movement in the War on Obesity

The term Health At Every Size has been used for years by a diverse group of people interested in deconstructing the prevailing narrative about weight and health. Researchers, clinicians, activists and others began to question the unexamined assumptions that people with a higher weight are always unhealthy and that weight loss always translates into improved health. This group eventually coalesced into the Association for Size Diversity and Health (ASDAH). Linda Bacon's paradigm-shifting book *Health at Every Size: The Surprising Truth about Your Weight* brought the term into more prominence.[1] Because of concerns that the phrase might be co-opted to support weight loss goals, ASDAH applied for and received registered trademarks for Health At Every Size and HAES in 2011 and 2012, respectively. The following is from the ASDAH website (www.sizediversityandhealth.org):

The Health At Every Size™ Principles*

1. **Weight Inclusivity:** Accept and respect the inherent diversity of body shapes and sizes and reject the idealizing or pathologizing of specific weights.
2. **Health Enhancement:** Support health policies that improve and equalize access to information and services and personal practices that improve human well-being, including attention to individual physical, economic, social, spiritual, emotional, and other needs.
3. **Respectful Care:** Acknowledge our biases and work to end weight discrimination, weight stigma, and weight bias. Provide information and services from an understanding that socioeconomic status, race, gender, sexual orientation, age, and other identities impact weight stigma, and support environments that address these inequities.
4. **Eating for Well-being:** Promote flexible, individualized eating based on hunger, satiety, nutritional needs, and pleasure, rather than any externally regulated eating plan focused on weight control.

---

*The terms Health At Every Size and HAES are trademarked by the Association for Size Diversity and Health and are used here with permission.

5. **Life-Enhancing Movement:** Support physical activities that allow people of all sizes, abilities, and interests to engage in enjoyable movement to the degree that they choose.

These principles guide the work that I do (and the way that I live my life). Let's look at some ways to apply them in moving toward a better relationship with food and eating and in valuing the bodies we have right now.

Getting Past the Dieting Mentality

When I talk of diets, I am referring to a deliberate effort to restrict food intake with the intent to lose weight. This can take many forms, from expensive commercial programs with preprepared foods, supplements, or weekly meetings to an eating plan found in a magazine, doctor's office, or online. Because the word *diet* has become associated with deprivation and discomfort, a popular alternative term is *lifestyle change*. Increasingly, I hear people say, "Oh, we all know that diets don't work. It's all about controlling portion sizes/avoiding junk food/eating healthy." There are countless variations on this theme.

If the intent is to lose weight, it is dieting mentality. If there is a "good food/bad food" dichotomy, it is dieting mentality. If there are rules to follow that result in feelings of guilt and shame when they are broken, it is dieting mentality.

Another term for this is *anorexic ideation*, which refers to the thought processes of those who struggle with anorexia nervosa, when the focus on weight loss has been carried to a life-threatening extreme. This may also be thought of as *eating disorder logic*, which incorporates all the assumptions about restricting intake, equating exercise with calorie burning, separating foods into acceptable versus unacceptable categories, etcetera. Whether we call it dieting mentality, anorexic ideation, or eating disorder logic, it is a problem.

Dieting mentality is so pervasive in our society that it is considered normal, especially for women. Disparaging comments about one's own body, weight, and eating are so common as to be unremarkable, but that does not negate the damage they cause. The assumption that weight loss is always a good thing is rarely questioned or challenged. Additionally, the assumption that the *focus* on weight loss is always a good thing is rarely questioned or challenged.

A paper by Mond et al. that was published in a public health journal came to an important conclusion:

When both the prevalence of BD (body dissatisfaction) and the degree of associated impairment are considered, it is apparent that there is a very substantial public health burden of BD at the population level. Hence, the present findings suggest that greater attention may need to be given to BD as a public health problem in its own right. . . . An additional implication of the present findings is that the fact that dissatisfaction with weight or shape is "normative" in industrialized nations should not be taken to infer that it is benign.[2]

Just because dieting mentality, anorexic ideation, and eating disorder logic are so pervasive that they are considered "normal" does not mean that they are harmless; indeed, they serve to perpetuate body dissatisfaction, anxiety, and disordered eating. Body dissatisfaction, and the unquestioning focus on weight loss that leads to it, can be considered "a public health problem in its own right."

How do we get past all that? The first step is to be aware of our own internal dialog and external commentary. This involves paying close attention to what we say to ourselves and to others. In this sense, dieting mentality is a habit that can be changed with effort, once it is recognized.

We are working toward improved quality of life and a better relationship with food and with our own bodies. For this to fully happen, the goal of weight loss has to be reconsidered. People who embrace a style of eating based on internal signals rather than a focus on weight loss find that their weight may drift upward, or downward, or it may stay the same, but their quality of life definitely improves.

As an example, Charlotte was a middle-aged lady who came to see me through her six-session employee assistance program (EAP) because she had heard from a friend about my approach to eating difficulties. She often binged and was generally unhappy about her eating and weight. She seemed to be very open to and interested in the information I discussed with her, but she made no progress. Finally, in the last session covered by her EAP, she admitted to me that this was "just an experiment" for her and that all along her plan was to go on yet another diet as soon as we used up her allotted sessions. She had not even attempted to let go of the dieting mentality and her intention to try to lose weight.

Before I go any further with suggestions for changing dieting mentality, I need to address a couple of concerns. If you have lived most of your life trying to follow a set of rules, you may want to turn my suggestions into a new set of rules. Please be aware of that and question any tendency to try to find a new set of hard-and-fast regulations to follow. Eating is very individual, and you get to adapt it to what works for you, understanding that it may change from day to day. In addition, some people have specific medical limitations on how they eat, whether it is for diabetes, congestive heart failure, phenylketonuria, celiac disease, or any other physical condition. If you have been diagnosed with a medical condition that limits your food choices, please continue to follow those guidelines. At the same time, if you have been told that weight loss will treat your medical issue, question that recommendation and do your own research.

You get to make your own decisions because of the Underpants Rule.

Why Do We Eat?

How often have I heard, "My problem is that I love to eat"? This statement is often followed by, "as you can tell by looking at me." Loving food is not the problem, nor is it possible to know how someone eats just by looking at them.

As human beings, we are hardwired to enjoy eating. It is a survival mechanism that helps keep the human race going. Sometimes when a person is depressed, sick, or receiving chemotherapy, she may lose pleasure in eating, which can quickly lead to dangerous weight loss. Eating is necessary to feed and nourish our bodies; if it is enjoyable at the same time, all the better!

One of the many common misconceptions about weight is that being overweight is caused by enjoying food too much and, therefore, consuming too much. This concept gets twisted into the idea that large people are not allowed to enjoy their food because the enjoyment will lead them to overeat and gain weight. Then it gets really complicated.

Part of the dieting mentality is the belief that "I shouldn't be eating at all, and I certainly shouldn't be enjoying it. I am not entitled to take pleasure in my food." This leads to several problematic behaviors, including (but not limited to) eating in secret, eating very quickly so as to avoid tasting anything that might be delicious, and limited satisfaction or satiety. Eating is then followed by guilt and shame, which leads to an increased effort to "be good."

In fact, considerable evidence exists to show that slowing down and truly savoring tasty food leads to *decreased* intake and improved nutrition. Eating food that we enjoy may even lead to improved absorption of important nutrients, such as iron, in the digestive system.[3]

Another misconception is that increased weight is related to "food addiction." The research on "food addiction" is questionable and contradictory. We are all born needing to eat. We are not addicted to food any more than we are addicted to water or sleep. The term *addiction* has come to be very loosely defined: some people claim to be "addicted" to television shows or social media, meaning that they are unhappy when they do not have it. The original definition of *addiction* refers to a physiological condition caused by the introduction of a substance to the body that results in the need for the substance, followed by increased tolerance and physical withdrawal symptoms. Some substances, such as caffeine, nicotine and alcohol, are addictive. Many others are not (see chapter 2 for more about the science behind the concept of food addiction).

Food is not addictive in this sense. Yes, certain foods that give us pleasure cause specific parts of the brain to light up on a brain scan, but those parts respond to other things that give us pleasure as well, such as the sight of a loved one or the sound of a baby laughing. When people say, "I am addicted to sugar (or chocolate or white flour or whatever), so I have to avoid it at all costs," they are setting themselves up for a sense of deprivation that can lead to preoccupation with that food and, possibly, a binge. This is altogether different from avoiding a certain food because you have paid attention to how you feel after eating it and do not like it. For instance, some individuals find that eating something high in sugar on an empty stomach results in a cranky headache an hour later, which is a valid reason to not do so.

Fueling our bodies is not the only reason we eat. We interact with food in many ways for many reasons. We use food preparation as a way of showing value and expressing affection when we take cookies to a new neighbor or prepare a wonderful meal for a valued friend. When we take a casserole to a bereaved household, food can be comfort as well as nutrition. Food preparation can be a form of artistic expression that focuses on pleasing the senses of sight, smell, and touch as well as taste. We all deserve to enjoy these activities; we do not need to earn the right to use food for pleasure, comfort, or affection.

Eating and Self-Esteem

"I have low self-esteem. I know I should take better care of myself, eat better, and lose weight, but I just can't make myself. I have always had low self-esteem." When Sharon came to my office for the first time with this presenting problem, she had no idea how common these feelings are. The term *low self-esteem* has become a catchall term for many problems that impair quality of life.

Self-esteem is basically how we value ourselves. We begin learning what is valuable about us early in life from the messages and treatment we receive from parents, family members, teachers, and other people in our lives. If a child hears that she is smart, thoughtful, and compassionate, that is what she will believe about herself. If she hears that she is ugly, stupid, and worthless, then that is what she will believe about herself. If she is occasionally told that she is special but is often neglected, she learns that she is unimportant. If she is only told that she is pretty, she will believe that prettiness is her only valuable attribute.

As we grow up, our feelings of self-esteem and self-worth are affected by what we hear from our peers, our significant others, and from the society in which we live. When we live in a culture that places enormous value on looking a certain way, it is understandable that we focus on physical "flaws" in ourselves and each other. In particular, current Western culture values thinness to an extreme degree; not only are we affected ourselves, but the people we look to for feedback are also affected. The message "You are too fat" is everywhere.

It is understandable, then, that a common way to try to improve self-esteem is to try to lose weight. Unfortunately, as we have already seen, attempts to lose weight almost always end in weight regain, which then contributes to the sense of failure that further erodes self-esteem.

How, then, do we improve self-esteem?

The Message We Give Ourselves

Some years ago, an advertisement for an expensive hair color product used the slogan "Because I'm worth it." How can we apply that idea of "I'm worth it" to eating and self-esteem?

When Sharon blamed her lack of self-care on her low self-esteem, she was surprised when I suggested she had it backward. She, like many others, felt that she had to feel good about herself to take good care of herself. Instead, I encouraged her to take good care of herself first, so that, over time, she learned to value herself more.

Think of it this way: if someone you care about deeply is coming to your house for dinner, you are probably going to invest some time and energy into fixing an appealing meal. We commonly use food to communicate, "You are important to me." We use food to say, "I value you," every time we take a casserole to a sick friend or cookies to a new neighbor. We can do that for ourselves, too.

You have several opportunities every day to tell yourself what you think you are worth. If you eat your lunch out of a piece of paper in one hand while driving the car or working at the computer with the other hand, you are giving yourself a message about what you think you are worth. If you really like Big Macs, then go to the drive-through window, get the sandwich, go home, unwrap it, put it on a plate, throw away the paper, sit at the table, light a candle, turn on some music, and enjoy your meal; you are now giving yourself a very different message about what you think you are worth. If you are able to go to the store, buy some ground beef, cheese, lettuce, tomato, and buns, go home and fire up the grill or stove and enjoy your cheeseburger at the table, you are giving yourself yet another message about what you think you are worth. The nutritional value changes very little, but the emotional nurturance is quite dissimilar.

Sharon, who lived alone, said, "But why would I go to all that trouble just for me?" Why wouldn't she? Each time she takes the time to fix a tasty meal just for herself, her self-esteem will improve because she is beginning to believe she is worth it. She had been willing to cook elaborate meals for her children and husband, but she snacked on convenience foods once the children were grown and she and her husband divorced. The concept that she was just as deserving of a nice meal when by herself was startling to her. She agreed to experiment with some slow cooker recipes, which she enjoyed reading about on social media but never tried, so that she would have a lovely aroma and a delicious dinner to welcome her home after a long day at work.

One of the unintended impacts of the focus on weight loss is the sense that we are not entitled to enjoy our food. This is partly because of the mistaken idea that people get fat because they enjoy food too much. This can then be internalized as a fear that enjoying food will lead to overeating. Instead, taking the time to really taste the flavors, revel in the textures, and mindfully take pleasure in eating usually results in more satisfaction with the amount of food that is just right for your body at that moment.

The dieting mentality includes a thought process that any eating at all is questionable, but eating anything that is tasty and delectable is forbidden. Thus, pleasurable eating is accompanied by guilt and shame. What effect does this have on self-esteem? Changing the pattern takes time and effort, but imagine what your self-esteem would be like if you approached every meal or snack with an attitude of "I deserve to enjoy this delicious food and feel good about myself afterward" and then did so?

Melissa is a middle-aged woman who lives with her disabled mother. She related to me that she left work and went home every day on her lunch break to check on her mother, and she implied to her coworkers that she ate lunch with her mother. She let her mother think that she ate lunch with her coworkers. In reality, she went to a drive-through window at a fast food place each day and then ate very quickly in the car where no one could see her. When she told me about this, her sense of shame about it was palpable. Because she had always been fat, she felt that she was not entitled to eat at all and was terrified by the possibility of criticism from her mother or coworkers. After she was finally able to confess this to me, we talked about eating as a way to improve self-esteem, and she was able to commit to some changes. While eating with her mother was still a challenge, she began taking the fast food back to her workplace to eat it at a table in the break room. When she gave herself permission to eat all the fast food she wanted without shame, she discovered that she did not like it as much as she thought! Eventually, she felt enough better about herself that she found the motivation to pack a lunch of food that she enjoyed and eat it in the company of her work friends.

Sometimes circumstances compel us to eat in the car rather than not eating at all; when that happens, eat without shame. Whenever possible, though, eat at a table from dishes that do not get thrown away afterward. Take food out of the package or carton and eat it from a washable dish; if you want more, give yourself permission to get more. Self-esteem improves when you treat yourself as if you are "worth it."

There is a difference between guilt and shame, but both are crippling to good self-esteem. Essentially, guilt is "I did something bad," while shame is "I am bad." Sometimes a feeling of guilt may be appropriate, but unreasonable, unrelenting guilt can easily become a soul-crushing sense of shame.

Feeling guilty about eating is so common in our culture that it passes unnoticed. That does not make it okay. Advertisers use it to sell food, with phrases like "guilty pleasures" or "sinfully decadent." It pops up in lunchtime conversations when someone says, "I shouldn't eat this. I'm so bad!" Everyone else accepts the comment as ordinary, and some may even chime in with, "You're not as bad as me!"

Everyone needs to eat, so why should anyone feel bad about it? We feel that way because the dieting industry has taught us that as a way to increase their profits. When is it reasonable to feel guilty about eating? Perhaps you might feel guilty if you violate religious restrictions that have been voluntarily agreed to. If the food was stolen from the refrigerator in a common area at work or in a dormitory, eating it should probably be accompanied by guilt. However, feeling guilty about eating because your diet says you are not supposed to is eventually going to lead to shame and diminishing self-esteem.

One of the more toxic effects of the "war on obesity" is the idea that shaming people for their weight will motivate them to become thinner and, therefore, healthier. This idea is based, in part, on the fact that past public health initiatives based on shame have had good results in improving behavior when applied to drunk driving, wearing seat belts, or smoking tobacco. The difference, of course, is that all of those things are behaviors that can be changed, but weight is a characteristic. The research literature shows that people who feel good about themselves make better decisions about healthy behaviors than people who feel ashamed, regardless of their weight. Yet, the idea persists that shaming people about their weight is not only helpful but obligatory. (For more about this, see Susan Greenhalgh's excellent book *Fat-Talk Nation: The Human Costs of America's War on Fat*.)[4]

Letting go of guilt and shame about eating and weight is challenging in a culture that consistently reinforces it, but the benefits are considerable. Self-esteem improves, which leads to better self-care, increased confidence, expanded emotional health, and more pleasure in life. When we treat ourselves with compassion, we experience enhanced strength, resilience, and quality of life.

What message do you want to give yourself about your own worth when you eat? Eating something you do not really like over the sink while feeling shameful is a behavior you can change. Each time you eat something delicious in a relaxed, pleasant surrounding while focusing on your own enjoyment, your sense of worth increases. Each time you invest time and effort in preparing exactly what you want, exactly the way you want it, you give yourself a message about what you think you are worth. Each time you plan ahead to be sure that you have the food that you enjoy when you want it, you believe that you are worth it. Everyone has to eat to survive; each occasion of eating is a chance to feel good about yourself.

Goal Setting and Self-Esteem

The way we set and achieve goals has a considerable impact on our self-esteem. Success improves self-esteem, while failure erodes it. But how do we define success and failure? It is very easy to set goals in ways that guarantee failure. If we change the way we set goals, we are more likely to succeed and then feel good about ourselves.

The most obvious way to ensure failure is to set a goal that is clearly unachievable. "I'm going to be the prima ballerina for the Joffrey Ballet" is obviously an impossible goal if I am a middle-aged nondancer. It is usually easy to identify and avoid that kind of goal setting.

A less obvious way to ensure failure is to set a goal that cannot be measured. "I just want to be a better wife" is a goal that I hear occasionally. What does that mean? How will you know if you have achieved it? When will you measure it?

When I worked on inpatient psychiatric units, we wrote treatment plans for each patient and reviewed them regularly. We were required to write objectives that were specific, measurable, achievable, and time limited. For someone who was depressed, "Patient will cheer up" would not be an acceptable objective. However, "Patient will laugh spontaneously at least once per shift within seven days" would be.

If you want to be a better partner, an acceptable objective might be "I will greet my spouse with a kiss when arriving home from work at least three days per week" or "I will engage in conversation with my significant other for 30 minutes at a time with the television off and my phone in the other room at least four times a week." After a week, you can evaluate how well you did at meeting the objectives, and you will know whether you succeeded.

Another problem with goal setting is having goals that are so large that they are overwhelming. This is when objectives become important. Objectives are smaller and more manageable. Breaking down a goal into steps that can be easily pictured or imagined increases motivation and decreases anxiety.

Some years ago, when I worked in the hospital and led a group on goal setting, one gentleman was really struggling with this concept. "I want to get my life back on track!" was the only goal he could articulate. I knew he was a football fan, and so I came up with an analogy that I have used many times since, for myself as well as the people I work with. It goes like this: Imagine you are a high school football coach. It is the halfway through the second quarter, you are down 7 to 3, you have the ball on your own 40-yard line, and it is second and 10. What do you want your quarterback to be thinking about? Do you want him thinking about playing in the NFL? Do you want him thinking about a college scholarship to play football? Do you want him thinking about winning the state championship? About winning the game? About scoring a touchdown? Or do you want him thinking about the next 10 yards?

When feeling overwhelmed, it can be helpful to ask, "What is my next 10 yards?" Gloria came to see me for help with her pattern of binge eating followed by shame and restriction. Her goals of "Eat better" and "Take care of myself" were vague and daunting. When I challenged her to focus on the next 10 yards, she said, "Make a grocery list." She then made a list with my help—first and 10! Her next 10 yards was "Go to the grocery store and buy everything on the list." She did not need to think about cooking until she had accomplished the trip to the store. When she focused on one objective at a time, she calmly made progress toward her goal.

"I want to take better care of myself" seems like a good idea, but how do you break it down? How and when do you measure it? Good short-term objectives might include "I will walk for 30 minutes at least three days a week," "I will eat at least three fruits and vegetables per day at least three days a week," or "I will be in bed by 10:00 p.m. at least four nights a week." At the end of the week, you can clearly say whether you achieved them. If you discover that the objectives were too hard or too easy, you can adjust them for the following week. Consistently achieving goals contributes to improved self-esteem.

Another way that people regularly set goals that ensure failure is to make the goal contingent on someone else's behavior. "I want my boss to treat me better" is understandable, but you have no control over what your boss does. In fact, anytime we focus on another person's behavior, we generally end up feeling helpless and out of control. When we bring the focus back to our own behavior, the situation may not change very much, but our sense of being in control changes.

If a person goes to a job interview with the goal "I'm going to get the job," then the goal is based on the behavior of the person making the decision rather than the behavior of the applicant. If the goal is "I'm going to be well prepared, stay calm, answer the questions to the best of my ability, and dress appropriately," then the goal is achievable even if the job offer does not happen. Focusing on succeeding at doing well at the interview rather than the outcome of getting the job has an effect on self-esteem.

A basic behavioral principle that applies to goal setting involves the way the objective is worded. We get better results when we say what we want rather than what we do not want. For instance, "I'm going to stay calm" works better than "I won't get scared." It is easier to recognize what is wrong than to identify what to do instead; it seems to be human nature. Developing a habit of articulating the desired behavior instead is very useful. Saying, "I'm not going to diet or focus on weight loss anymore," is a good start, but what do you do instead? Alternate objectives include "I will eat at least three times a day, and I will eat a variety of foods" or "I will plan ahead so that I have food available when I get hungry."

There are certainly a lot of things in the world that we have no control over. Contrary to what we read and see in the media, we have very limited control over our weight (beyond causing it to increase by repeated attempts at weight loss dieting). We have no control over what other people do, but we have control over how we respond. We have limited control over our health, but we do have control over our health-related behaviors, such as smoking or physical activity. When we focus on achievable and measurable behavioral goals, we increase our chances of success, and we will see improved self-esteem as a result.

Goals based on the number on the scale are likely to erode self-esteem. Goals based on behaviors, such as engaging in enjoyable physical activity and consuming a variety of delicious foods, are likely to improve self-esteem.

Let's consider a goal of "I want to stop feeling bad about myself." First, how can you make it be about what you want rather than what you do not want? "I want to feel better about myself." This is clearly a desirable outcome, but it needs objectives that are measurable and behavioral. Objectives could include such things as "I will eat at least one meal a day that is food that I enjoy while sitting at a table with real dishes," "I will spend my afternoon break sitting outside in the sunshine at least three times this week," or "I will leave work in time to get to my yoga class on Tuesday, even if someone stops me with a question." How many times a day do you have an opportunity to give yourself the message that you are valuable? If you always wear your seat belt in the car, for instance, you can remind yourself each time you buckle up, "I'm worth it." If you do not wear your seat belt, can you consider it something you can do to remind yourself of your value?

Finally, take time to congratulate yourself each time you achieve an objective. It is easier to focus on what still needs to be done—again, this seems to be human nature—but behavior that is positively reinforced is more likely to happen again. When you accomplish an objective, pay attention. Sit with it for a moment. Feel good about what you have done. Consider writing down your objectives and setting a timeline for evaluating them. Give yourself credit for doing what you said you would do. Enjoy it!

Self-Compassion

It seems so much easier to feel compassion for others than for ourselves, yet we are more important to ourselves than anyone else is. In some ways, self-compassion is the opposite of shame. When we treat ourselves with compassion and gentleness, our strength increases, and our brittleness decreases. This is true when things are going well, but it is especially true when we make mistakes.

My yoga teacher often talks about "the story you tell yourself in your head." This is similar to the concepts in cognitive behavioral therapy, but I like the phrase "story you tell yourself" better. Thoughts are mental events that may or may not represent truth. How we shape our thoughts influences how we feel and behave, and we have a certain amount of control over our thoughts. First, we have to notice them. The tree pose in yoga involves standing on one foot and placing the bottom of the other foot against the standing leg. It sounds simple, but the balance involved is often challenging. It is tempting to think, "I can't believe I still can't do this! What is wrong with me?" My teacher often says something along the lines of, "Be aware of your thoughts. If this pose is not available to you today, that does not make you a bad person. If you put your big toe mound on the floor, it is still tree pose." This changes the story.

Self-compassion is more likely to lead to positive behavioral change than self-shaming. We only have one life to live, and we live it in the only body we are going to have. Being compassionate with ourselves and with our bodies moves us toward having the best life we can.

Relearning to Eat

The idea that the body cannot be trusted is the foundation of the dieting culture and the dieting industry. All diets are based on the belief that individuals will eat uncontrollably and gain weight unless they have guidelines from someone more knowledgeable. The concept that the body and its hungers are a source of useful information is then considered downright dangerous. This myth is what is dangerous! In chapter 2, the studies by Edholm and Sims, among others, demonstrated that the body can be trusted to manage its own energy balance without outside interference.[5,6]

If you have been dieting most of your life, a nondieting approach may seem scary. What do you do instead? There are different names for different approaches, such as intuitive eating, mindful eating, competent eating, and attuned eating, and they are all ways to learn to eat based on internal signals and trusting your body. Another related concept is about internal and external locus (or location) of control.

In the field of personality psychology, internal and external locus of control refers to our beliefs about what we have control over and what is beyond our control. Do we attribute outcomes in our lives to our own behaviors or to outside influences? The concept is applied to many different circumstances and variables, but I am interested in how it applies to decisions about eating.

Dieting is based on an external locus of control; essentially, it is the idea that I cannot make good decisions about what or how much to eat, so I have to have someone else tell me. One example of this is the marketing approach of 100-calorie packages of snack food. Who decided that a serving size of 100 calories is just right? What if I am really hungry? What if I only want 49 calories' worth? Why am I not competent to make that choice?

An external locus of control requires the belief that I am not capable of making those decisions—someone else will do a better job. How is it that Jenny Craig knows more about what I should be eating than I do?

An internal locus of control honors the body's appetites and needs. It involves listening to the body's signals. It requires asking questions: "Am I hungry? How hungry am I? What am I hungry for? Am I full yet? Does this food satisfy me? How do I feel after I eat it? When will I be ready to eat again?" Eating according to an internal locus of control involves asking these questions several times a day and deciding the best way to respond.

Clara was convinced that her diet was the only thing standing between her and uncontrollable bingeing. The idea of eating according to an internal locus of control was frightening, but a future of shame-filled dieting was even more frightening. Like many other women who have worked with me, she had a few episodes of overeating after she made a commitment to eat according to her internal cues, but she then found that she did not know her own preferences as well as she thought. When she gave herself permission to eat whatever she wanted, as much as she wanted, her appetite normalized, and she began to feel hungry for fruits and vegetables as well as previously "forbidden" foods. Then came the day when she sadly told me, "Cheesecake just doesn't taste as good as I've imagined all these years!"

Trust your body; it knows what it is doing. Dieting or eating according to an external locus of control erodes self-trust. If we cannot trust ourselves to make choices about what we eat, what can we trust ourselves to make choices about?

Cindy came to me because of conflict with her boss and because "I see you work with eating disorders." After a bad day at the office (which was practically every day), she would go home and binge. She was well and truly tired of the diet rollercoaster and embraced the idea of eating according to an internal locus of control. She began eating better at lunch and breakfast, her bingeing stopped, and then she surprised herself: she stood up for herself to her boss, who then began treating her better!

Cindy's story did not surprise me; I had seen similar situations before. People who felt great uncertainty in other areas of their lives found more confidence when they began to trust themselves to make decisions about eating. When they practiced self-trust several times a day about food, they developed more assurance in other areas, and they were able to be more assertive in relationships.

Learning to trust yourself about food choices takes time and practice, and there will be mistakes along the way. Mistakes are a chance to learn. Be gentle with yourself. Initially, it may be helpful to have a meal plan as a guideline. There is a big difference between a diet and a meal plan: the focus of a diet is "Don't eat too much!" The focus of a meal plan is "Be sure to eat enough!" The most basic meal plan includes at least three meals a day, at least five servings of complex carbohydrates, at least five servings of fruits and vegetables, at least three servings of high-quality protein, and at least a couple of servings of dairy each day. If you want more, that's fine—have more. If you eat that much, then when you encounter a previously forbidden food, you will be more likely to eat a reasonable amount rather than bingeing because you will not be overly hungry. The meal plan is a temporary step in the journey for relearning to eat according to internal cues that you can use as long as you need to and can come back to if you have difficulties in the future.

In chapter 1, I used the example of a sleep-deprived college student to demonstrate the idea that physiological processes cannot be overcome through "willpower." Kathy Kater outlines a wonderful experiential activity for grade schoolers called "The Air Diet" in her curriculum *Healthy Bodies*.[7] In it, the teacher playfully suggests that the youngsters have been "breathing too much" and issues straws to breathe through to limit air intake. After a couple of minutes, when they are allowed to breath normally again, they gasp for air and are asked why they are "overbreathing." This illustrates that the normal physiological response to being deprived of our basic need for breathing results in taking big gulps of air, just as restrictive eating often results in gulping food.

Binge eating is almost always preceded by undereating. People who do not diet do not binge. Physically, dieting keeps a person in a perpetual state of hunger. Psychologically, dieting teaches a person to expect a period of restriction after any time of unrestricted eating. The way to avoid binge-ing is to follow a meal plan that ensures adequate intake. Everyone has food cravings at least occasionally. Restricted eating combined with crav-ings usually leads to a binge, while eating according to an internal locus of control can accommodate cravings with ease. The meal plan eventually becomes unnecessary as your body learns to trust in regular, adequate nutrition.

A phrase that has become more common in the last few years is *food inse-curity*. Initially, it was used to refer to households and families where access to adequate food was limited by low income. It is an important social policy consideration. When a family is on food stamps, for instance, they usually develop a pattern of ending the month with limited or no food, followed by an influx of groceries after the first of the month with behavior that is similar to bingeing. This is an expectable, understandable response to food scarcity, but it raises the concern that children who grow up with this pattern may lose their ability to recognize hunger and fullness in an ordinary way and are vulnerable to disordered eating patterns. This is similar to dieting mentality. The fear that food will not be available in the future makes it very difficult to eat reasonably in the present, a pattern that may persist long after the food insecurity is resolved.

How do we evaluate progress? (Remember when we talked about goal setting?) If you were binge eating before, have you stopped or reduced the frequency? This involves an honest measurement; how often were you bingeing before? Bingeing is defined as eating a large amount of food with an accompanying sense of loss of control. The goal is not to reduce the amount eaten but to reduce the feeling of loss of control. Let me repeat that: the goal is to reduce the feeling of loss of control. Feeling out of control is very unpleasant and can be avoided by learning to eat from an internal locus of control.

Another measure of progress is a subjective observation of your own thoughts. I often ask people how much time they spend thinking about food. The answer is frequently, "All the time!" or "Ninety-five percent of the day!" Those answers indicate a pattern of undereating and restriction. I then ask, "What would it be like to only think about food 30 or 40 percent of the time?" The answer is usually enthusiastically positive. People who are not trying to lose weight usually think about food only 30–40 percent of the time, when they are hungry or planning meals (unless they work in food service). That allows 60–70 percent of the day to think about other things. What would you be thinking about if you were not thinking about food?

Dieting can often be an effective distraction from other life stressors. It gives the illusion of control. When we feel out of control with life circumstances, we often try to find a body-oriented solution. When we feel anxious about our jobs, our marriages, or our finances, we can find temporary relief by focusing on trying to make our bodies smaller. However, when we try to manage emotional dysregulation by dieting, we then add physical dysregulation and hunger, which then backfires, adding an additional sense of shame to whatever else is going badly. Sometimes the focus on the sense of failure itself is an effective distraction from other distressing concerns. Giving up dieting may mean having to notice all the other problems in life. What would you be thinking about or worrying about if you were not focused on dieting?

Self-compassion also includes recognizing that whatever you have been doing with food or food avoidance, it is because, at some point, the behavior served a purpose for you. It is not necessary to feel bad about what you have been doing to find a way that works better.

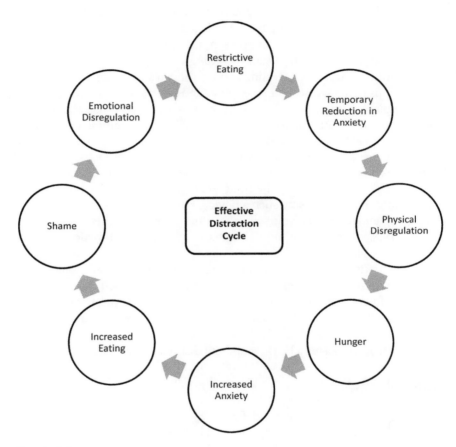

Figure 3.1

Quantifying and Measuring

Measuring outcomes is an important part of evaluating behavior, but it carries the potential to become a problem in and of itself. Finding a balance between flexibility and achievement can be tricky, especially for people who have a long history of diet mentality and external locus of control. One way to check this is to ask, "How is this helping? How is it hurting?" Meeting your goals should feel good. If, instead, you notice a sense of failure, then it is time to reevaluate. Sometimes the goals were too ambitious, and sometimes circumstances change. Whatever the reason, this process should produce feelings of improved self-worth; tweak accordingly.

Personally, I have mixed feelings about the various fitness trackers and wellness apps that have become so popular and prevalent. I have seen numerous examples of improved physical activity when people use them, but I worry about how easily the technology can backfire and reinforce feelings of failure. Using a device to track behavior may start out as a tool, but when does it become another method of relying on an external locus of control? When does it begin to undermine trust in one's own bodily experience? At what point does the focus on the numbers interfere with autonomous decision making? If you are using such a device, evaluating its usefulness may be an ongoing endeavor. Ask yourself, from time to time, "Is this helping? Is it hurting? How does it make me feel better about myself? How does it make me feel worse about myself?"

I was recently in a social situation where several middle-aged women were discussing their fitness trackers. One said that she skipped her lunchtime walk if she forgot her tracker "because it wouldn't count." Another shared her idea of tying her tracker to her shoelace at the grocery store because it did not register her steps when her hands were stationary on the shopping cart. Somehow, it seems easy to let the numbers distract from the original intent.

"You Must Be Present to Win"

The concept of mindfulness is defined by Jon Kabat-Zinn as "paying attention in a particular way: on purpose, in the present moment, and nonjudgmentally."[8] Intuitive eating, defined by Tylka,[9] includes three components: (1) unconditional permission to oneself to eat when hungry and to eat the desired food; (2) eating for physical reasons rather than emotional reasons; and (3) reliance on internal hunger and satiety cues to decide what, when, and how much to eat. Intuitive, or mindful, eating is associated with improved physical health, improved psychological well-being, and less disordered eating. It relies on an internal locus of control for making decisions about food.

How do we embrace being nonjudgmental? This is tricky for just about everyone. Negative internal evaluation seems to be the default; being nonjudgmental takes effort and awareness. One component of mindfulness is simply being aware of your own thoughts. Notice how often your evaluation of yourself is negative. What would it feel like to change those judgments to neutral curiosity?

Danny is a young man who originally came to see me for treatment of his anxiety. One of the ways he had tried to deal with it on his own was by channeling his energy into extremely restrictive eating. Restoring adequate nutrition helped some, and then we were able to talk about his internalized negative dialog. When talking with me about how he felt, he frequently prefaced his comments with, "This is going to sound stupid" or "You're going to think this is stupid." When I encouraged him to explore the feelings associated with these statements, he identified that he had been this way for years as a way to deflect criticism from his family. It had become a habit, a default way of thinking. However, it had not been helpful in deflecting criticism, and now it was contributing to his anxiety and constant fear of failure.

I encouraged Danny to notice his thoughts and be curious about them, to ask himself, "Hmm, it is interesting that those pesky thoughts have popped up again. I wonder what that is about?" As a result, he has increased his ability to self-observe, challenge, and change his self-deprecating thoughts. His anxiety has lessened, and his assertiveness at work has improved. His use of the word *stupid* has diminished dramatically.

Nonjudgmental attention is part of mindfulness meditation. Thoughts flit across the mind; notice them and let them go without judgment. A friend helped me understand this when she described part of her own meditation practice when focusing on her breath. She narrated it as, "Rising, falling, rising, falling, rising, falling, fretting, worrying. No! No! No! Rising, falling." She was able to change it to, "Rising, falling, rising falling, rising, falling. I'm fretting, worrying. Let it go. Rising, falling." The ability to notice her own intrusive thoughts and let them go without judgment helped her quiet her mind.

How Do You Feel?

Once you are able to sort out the thoughts that come from a dieting mentality, you can begin identifying how you feel. This is an ongoing process. A good way to start is by paying attention to what physical sensations follow eating certain foods or in certain ways. For instance, some people notice that if they eat a tasty, sugary food, an hour later they feel sluggish or headachy. Other people do not have that reaction. Some people experience a feeling of well-being after eating ice cream, while folks who struggle with lactose intolerance experience gastric distress. Everyone is different; the best way to learn your own patterns is by paying attention with curiosity and without judgment. Experiment with different ways of eating and then ask "How do I feel?" after you eat a certain food, and how you feel an hour or several hours later. For instance, if you are in the habit of eating a cup of yogurt for breakfast, you may notice that you feel satisfied at the time but become overly hungry before lunchtime. You can then try eating more for breakfast or adding a midmorning snack (if your situation allows) and observe the difference.

Sometimes it is tricky to sort out what you are actually feeling from what dieting has conditioned you to expect. For example, you may have avoided entrees with cream sauce at your favorite Italian restaurant because dieting mentality says they are "fattening." Now that all foods are allowed, you order one for dinner. You may find that (1) it is absolutely delicious; (2) it tastes yummy but you experience indigestion later; (3) you feel fine until you go to bed, when you experience acid reflux; (4) you are disappointed because it does not taste as good as you remember; or (5) you enjoy it, feel fine, order it the next three times you eat there, and then notice that you miss the pasta primavera that you used to order, so you get that instead. There are no right answers, just additional information about yourself, your preferences, and your body.

The question "Am I hungry?" is complicated, especially for those who have a history of restrained eating. How is hunger defined? Is it a growling in the stomach? Does it have to include lightheadedness and dizziness to qualify as hunger that deserves to be fed? Is it an awareness that eating might be a good idea? Relearning hunger awareness can take time and attention, too.

It can help to rate hunger on a low-to-high range. Different versions of such scales can be found in books or online, I have included my own here. If it does not work for you, feel free to use it as a guideline to come up with one for yourself.

Hunger Scale

1. My vision is blurry, and I am lightheaded and about to faint.
2. I need to eat right now!
3. I am famished. I should have thought about what to eat sooner.
4. It is time to eat, before my stomach starts to rumble.
5. This is really good.
6. Hmm, I wonder if I should take some of this home to have for lunch tomorrow?
7. Oh, that is so nice, just right! (I wonder if they have mints at the checkout?)
8. Okay, that was three bites too many.
9. This is so good, but I should have stopped eating five minutes ago.
10. I am so stuffed that I am afraid if I move I will barf!

Ideally, the goal is to stay close to the middle of the range, eating before you get to 3 and stopping before you get to 8. If you have been following an external locus of control, it may be difficult to judge this at first. Initially, eating by the clock can be helpful in learning your own hunger signals. Dieting creates a pattern of restricting followed by letting go, which results in psychological and physical expectations of deprivation. Following a meal plan that focuses on *enough* to eat on a predictable, dependable schedule helps reset trust, in both body and mind, in sufficient and reliable nutrition. Once the body and the brain become confident that access to food will not be suddenly withdrawn, actual hunger will become easier to identify. Consistent, adequate nutrition makes listening to body cues much easier.

The concept of scarcity is used as a marketing tool. If availability of an item is limited, sales increase. The most familiar example of this is Girl Scout Cookies. We have all known people who become frantic if they cannot find a friend or coworker with a daughter or niece to buy cookies from during the limited time they are available. Sometimes people buy them to put in the freezer, only to eat them up before someone else can. The sense that "I have to get as much as I can while I can" drives up sales. If Girl Scout Cookies were available year-round, they probably would not sell as well. This applies to any food item that is "available for a limited time only," whether it is Easter candy or McRib sandwiches.

This concept of scarcity contributes to patterns of problematic eating choices. If you have internalized the concept that a certain food is forbidden or off limits, when that food becomes available, it becomes very difficult to stop eating it. The idea that "Once I finish this, I can never have it again" can make it impossible to maintain a sense of control. In contrast, when everything is allowed, it is possible to think, "Hmm, do I want this or not?"

Some years ago, I attended a community workshop on disaster response that was organized by the local police department. Next to the registration table was an enormous box of doughnuts. My first thought when I saw it was, "How did they even get that here? The box is too big to fit into a standard car!" I looked them over. However, I had eaten a good breakfast, and they were not the kind of doughnuts I like, so I got some coffee and sat down. I wondered how many people in the room would have a hard time listening to the speakers because they were so distracted by that huge box; the internalized idea that "Doughnuts are a bad food, so I can't have any"; and the overwhelming desire to eat them all.

Dieting as an Illusion of Control

No one likes to feel out of control. (Think of the last time you were in a car that was sliding on ice.) There are some things in life that we can control and many things that we cannot. When we feel out of control, we may focus on a body solution, as we discussed earlier. When distressing things happen in our lives, whether it has to do with work, relationships, finances, or anything else, we experience emotional dysregulation. A focus on what to eat or not eat in an attempt to control the body may provide a brief feeling of being in control, but it is an illusion. Attempting to reregulate emotional dysregulation by restricting intake adds physical dysregulation, which leads to hunger and preoccupation with food.

Dieting serves as a very effective distraction. If a woman is upset because her husband is staying out late, or her teenager won't clean her room, or her boss is demeaning, it is easy to focus instead on restrictive eating and weight loss. When her attempts inevitably fail, she can then focus on her feelings of guilt, shame, and worthlessness. The very unpleasantness of the pattern is an effective distraction from the real problems in her life and her sense of futility in addressing them.

Letting go of detrimental eating patterns may lead to an increase in anxiety when the other issues become impossible to ignore. It is a necessary step in identifying what problems need to be addressed and making a plan to address them. Again, consider the question: what would you be thinking or worrying about if you were not focused on food?

Worry, anxiety, and anger are uncomfortable, but they are survivable. Focusing on eating, not eating, and related distractions can divert us from whatever needs attending to. Which brings us to emotional eating.

Emotional Eating

Now I eat my feelings sometimes, but they're positive feelings, so they taste like vegetables and mostly happen at mealtimes.

—L. S. Quinn, comment on the "Health at Every Size" Facebook page

Emotional eating is a term, like many others, that is often used but rarely defined. It is usually considered to be a negative behavior, something that is irrational and shameful and that leads to weight gain. What happens if we try to approach this concept from a neutral perspective? What do we mean by the term as well as the behavior involved?

Food can fill an emotional need at the same time that it fills a nutritional need. We can be upset and hungry, too. Books and articles that focus on "weight management" or weight loss usually recommend paying attention to feelings as a way to delay or avoid eating because the goal is to eat less by any means available. We have already seen how that approach can backfire in ways both behavioral and psychological. Paying attention to feelings is a good practice all the time, not just when food is involved.

Feelings Are Normal

How do we define *normal*? My favorite definition is, "The setting on the clothes dryer between permanent press and high."

Everyone has feelings. Emotions are a normal part of the human experience. We can tolerate them, make space for them, and be curious and compassionate about them.

Just as with food, there is risk in categorizing emotions into good versus bad. Emotions and feelings simply are. Experiencing feelings may range from comfortable to uncomfortable, but they are not, in and of themselves, good or bad. When we label a feeling as bad and try to avoid it, we risk bottling it up and suppressing it until it builds into something dangerous and scary.

Theoretically, all feelings fall into one of four categories (with some overlap). Feelings can be angry, happy, sad, or scared. We tend to think of happy feelings as good and all the others as bad. However, the other feelings are appropriate as well, even if they are uncomfortable. Although we do not have much control over what we feel, we do have control over how we behave.

Let's take anger, as an example. Anger is a signal to ourselves that something is wrong and needs to be addressed. Anger can provide us with the energy we need to do what needs to be done. Trying to avoid feeling anger can result in an outburst (much as avoiding eating can result in a binge). Perhaps you have a coworker who regularly interrupts you in meetings and takes credit for your work. If you try to pretend to yourself that you are not annoyed, you risk having the anger fester and build until you have an inappropriate outburst in front of the entire staff. If, instead, you deal with the feeling when it is still small, you can make better choices; perhaps you talk with the coworker in private about the behavior and follow up with the boss if that does not work. Even if the outcome is not ideal, the anger is smaller and more manageable.

Having a larger vocabulary for feelings can help. Mental health professionals have a term for not having enough words for feelings: *alexithymia*. *A* means none, *lexi* means words, and *thymia* means feelings—having no words for your feelings. If you are experiencing uncomfortable emotions, having accurate labels engages a part of the brain that helps you feel more in control so you can think more clearly.

If you think that alexithymia may be a problem for you, a useful exercise is to make a list of all the words you can think of for each of the four categories of feelings: angry, happy, sad, and scared. See how long a list you can make on your own, then use a thesaurus. Now rank order them in terms of size and intensity. For instance, a small word for scared is *startled*, a big word is *terrified*. Keep the list handy so that you can refer to it when you are having trouble identifying exactly how you feel.

Focusing on food and eating, or focusing on limiting food and eating, are both effective short-term ways to avoid feeling uncomfortable emotions, but it ultimately impairs your ability to improve your well-being. Laura came to see me for help with her binge eating. She had a full-time job plus a husband and three teenagers, none of whom picked up after themselves. She felt that her house and her life were out of control, and her pattern was to try to achieve a sense of control by going on yet another diet. When she focused on what and how much she was going to eat, or not eat, she could avoid thinking about the troublesome parts of her life. Sooner or later, her hunger and deprivation resulted in a binge, and then she could focus on feeling guilt and shame while planning the next diet. This made it possible to ignore how angry she was with her family. Giving up the cycle of diet followed by guilt about breaking the diet meant she would have to deal with the issues in her life directly.

It is a natural human tendency to turn to eating for comfort. There is nothing wrong with this, as long as it does not stop us from doing what else we need to do. If the concept of *emotional eating* means that we should not eat when we are emotional, then it is another rule based on an external locus of control. Using an internal locus of control allows us to use a different set of questions: "Am I upset? What about? What are better words to describe how I feel?" We can also ask, "Do I need to eat something before I try to figure this out?" If you are hungry, your ability to think clearly is impaired. If you are not hungry, eating something may help you to calm down enough to think through how you feel and what to do next. Avoiding eating anything at all will likely increase your sense of being dysregulated.

If you decide you are going to use eating to self-sooth, make it count! Trying to make do with something "good for you" is probably not going to be as effective as eating what you really want (within the limits of what you already know about how your body reacts to specific foods). What food is going to best suit your needs in the moment? Is it possible to get that food? If not, what is the closest you can manage? Once you have it, take the time to enjoy and savor it, without guilt or question. Then you can move on to what needs to be done next.

Knowing what your comfort foods are and having them available saves time and energy that you can then use to address the questions that remain. What else are you hungry for? Companionship? Time alone? Encouragement? Talking with a particular person? How can you meet those needs? These questions are easier to answer with a comforted stomach. Additionally, you are giving yourself the message that you deserve to be soothed when you are upset.

Sometimes these steps can be combined. I often see people in my practice who are struggling with grief. Connecting around a memory of a favorite food is very comforting. Angie came to see me after losing her beloved grandmother. In response to my questioning, she identified that her grandmother loved fish sandwiches from a local restaurant. Even though fish sandwiches were not Angie's favorite, she found that getting one for herself and eating it at the park close to her grandmother's house gave her a sense of connection that she had been unable to find elsewhere. Similarly, Luanne began keeping carrot and celery sticks in the refrigerator in the plastic container that her mother had used for the same purpose before her death. She was able to use the vegetables to meet her physical nutrition needs as well as for finding comfort in her sadness. Most people would probably not think of carrots and celery as "comfort food," but they were for Luanne.

Contrary to the rules about dieting, there is nothing wrong with "comfort foods," unless they become an excuse to avoid doing what needs to be done. Sometimes diet rules include instructions to get comfort foods out of the house to avoid them. I recommend the opposite. Make sure you have what you want available when possible or something close if not possible. For instance, I will never have my grandmother's wonderful homemade egg noodles again, but I keep a package of Amish egg noodles in my pantry because they come very close. Because they are easily available, I can ask myself, "Is eating noodles what I really want, or do I need to call a friend/do some yoga/take a nap?"

If the comfort food is not available, the substitute will work better if it is as close as possible. This may require keeping a container of premium ice cream in the freezer for the times you want a Blizzard when Dairy Queen is closed and store-brand frozen vanilla yogurt just won't cut it. Remember, when you know that the ice cream is always available without restriction, bingeing behavior stops.

It may be necessary to make choices based on financial limitations. Sometimes what we want is simply too expensive to keep on hand. When this happens, be very clear in your awareness that the decision is based on money and not on calories, fat grams, or personal worth.

Dieting logic teaches that eating for emotional reasons is always bad. While I agree that sorting out feelings is vital, it is essential to be well nourished to do so. It is entirely possible to be upset and hungry at the same time, which makes understanding the feelings difficult, if not impossible. Taking a moment to have a satisfying snack or meal before trying to address the feelings improves your ability to figure it out.

Rebound Feelings

Disordered eating is an effective distraction from life's difficulties. Letting go of dieting and weight loss frees up time and energy, but it may also bring the world into sharper focus. Problems and difficulties that have been obscured by a preoccupation with not eating are suddenly visible and painful. When Melinda, a health care worker, finally got her bulimia under control, she complained to me that now she could no longer overlook all the unfairness and sadness in the world.

On the other hand, the world may become more vivid. Years ago, I met a very interesting, very large woman at an eating disorder conference, and she shared an poignant story with me. After years of failed dieting, she had been working on an assembly line and got laid off. When she was called back to work, she was told she was too heavy to be rehired, so she decided to have weight loss surgery. The evaluation for the surgery concluded that she was not fat enough to qualify (this was years ago, when the requirements were more stringent). She then decided to eat whatever she wanted in an attempt to gain weight to qualify. She told me something like this: "The most amazing thing happened. Not only did I feel better, but colors got brighter. Blues were bluer, greens were greener. Dieting reduced my life to shades of gray, and I never even realized it." She then gave up dieting forever, went back to school, and became an advocate for size acceptance.

This process can be heartrending. The recognition of the years of wasted time and effort in the futile attempt to become acceptably smaller can lead to anger, sadness, and grief. While uncomfortable, these feelings are survivable and may be a source of energy to make changes. Remember to breathe, find accurate labels for the feelings, take good care of yourself, and consider finding someone to help you talk it through. If you find that relinquishing dieting as a coping mechanism leaves you with intolerable anxiety, sadness or anger, it may be a good idea to find a mental health professional to help you. Counseling is another way you can give yourself a message that you are worth it (see chapter 10).

Suffering is optional is a concept from Buddhism that I find helpful personally as well as in my counseling practice. This is how I understand it: when we invest energy in wishing that things were different, we make ourselves miserable. We have a certain amount of control over whether we do so. I live in Missouri, so the example I often use is snow. During a snowstorm, some people stand in the window, looking out, and say, "Why is it snowing? I want it to stop snowing! This is ruining everything! Why won't it stop snowing?" They have no control over the snow, but they do have some control over how miserable they make themselves by investing energy in wishing that it was different. This is not to say that we should do nothing about things that can and need to change; it is about shifting where we invest our energy. Can you refocus your energy away from wishing that things were different and toward changing what you can?

CHAPTER FOUR

Eating 2.0: Upgrading Your Relationship with Food

What does it mean to eat well? To eat healthy? To eat normally? Everyone seems to have an opinion, and all the information found in any one place is contradicted somewhere else. It is rare to find someone who does not have views about how eating should happen and accompanying anxiety when those views are not followed. The conflicting rules, attitudes, opinions, and views hinder our ability to have a reasonable relationship with food.

Let's change the question. Instead of "What is good eating?" we can ask, "What does it mean to have a good relationship with food?" or, better yet, "What does it mean *for me* to have a good relationship with food?" Only you can answer that, but here are some ideas to consider:

- Eat when hungry; stop when full.
- Eat a wide variety of foods.
- Enjoy the act of eating.
- Sometimes eat foods that are not particularly enjoyable because there is nothing else available to nourish oneself.
- Think about food when hungry or when it is mealtime, and think about other things the rest of the time.
- Eat often enough to prevent feeling starved.
- Sometimes eat for reasons other than hunger.
- Allow for flexibility and spontaneity.
- Trust your body to know what it needs.

Having a good relationship with food is not going to happen overnight, especially if you have a long history of trying to change your body through restrictive eating, but it is certainly something you can work toward over time. Consider making a list of your own and adding to it or changing it as you go.

Good Foods/Bad Foods

The lists of good foods and bad foods have different names, but they are similar lists. Whether they are called *red light/green light* foods, *on program/off program* foods, or *healthy/unhealthy* foods, they are essentially the same. Anything that is tasty, appealing, and high in calories is bad, and anything low in calories is good. A variation on this is *eating clean*, the opposite of which is, obviously, *eating dirty*. Another is *eat right*, so any deviation from the instructions is, by definition, *eating wrong*. Any list that incorporates the idea that you should feel virtuous or shameful depending on what you eat is problematic. The more rules there are, the more likely you are to break them and then experience feelings of guilt and shame.

All foods are good foods, unless you are allergic to them. If a food makes you break out in hives, it is a bad food for you. Also, if it is spoiled, it is a bad food. Aside from that, some foods are more nutrient dense, some are more energy dense, and some are both. Vegetables generally have a lot of vitamins and minerals but not much energy. Candy has energy but not much else in the way of other nutrients. Steak has energy and also protein and iron. Foods that are high in nutrients but low in energy are generally categorized as *good foods*, but it may be challenging to eat enough of them to get sufficient energy.

Let's talk for a minute about that much maligned item, the *calorie*. I have often asked people to define *calorie* for me. I have received many answers, from a tentative "Calories are . . . um . . . bad?" to an authoritative "Calories are a measure of how good or bad a food is for you!" And now I have to share a story. My daughter, as an undergraduate, took a nutrition class in nursing school as part of her general education requirements. At one point, the instructor called on her. "Ms. Ordway, as the only physics major in this class, can you tell us what a calorie is?" She answered, "A calorie is a measure of energy. It is the amount of heat it takes to raise 1 gram of water 1 degree centigrade. But I didn't learn that in physics; I learned it from my mom." The instructor, startled, asked, "What does your mom do? Is she a physicist?"

Calories are a way of measuring how much energy the body accesses through intake. Some foods are densely packed with energy, such as butter, while others have almost none, such as watermelon. How much energy does a person need in a day? Probably more than you think. The current culture of the pursuit of thinness promotes an unending restriction of caloric intake; however many calories you are eating, it is considered too many. As a result, most people underestimate how many calories they need. In the Keys study (see chapter 2), 1,570 calories per day was considered starvation.[1] Per day, 1,570 calories is considerably more than most weight loss diets.

The largest part of our daily energy need, 60–75 percent, is simply for our basal metabolic rate (BMR), the amount needed for the body to function at rest. BMR is determined by genetics, age, body composition, and other factors. The average number of calories needed for BMR for adults is about 1,500, still more than many diets. Restrictive eating lowers the BMR by making it more efficient. (Think of your furnace or car: when you do something to make it more efficient, you get more heat or miles driven for less fuel.) All activity, even tossing and turning in your sleep, requires more energy in addition to the BMR.

Calories are an important part of our intake. We need enough calories every day for life to continue. Even food considered *empty calories* still contributes to our energy needs. While it might be possible, with effort, to put together an intake of less than 1,500 calories per day that still included sufficient vitamins, minerals, protein, carbohydrates, and lipids, it would still have insufficient energy. Human beings may develop other health complications without enough vitamins, minerals, or protein, but chronic inadequate calorie intake leads to starvation and death. Calories are necessary.

Meanwhile, our bodies have exquisitely well-developed mechanisms for adjusting our intake to exactly what we need. Much like the thermostat on our furnace that monitors the temperature and automatically turns on and off to maintain the setting, our hunger tells us when our energy needs to be replaced, and our fullness indicates sufficient intake. While we may need to pay attention to getting enough nutrient-dense foods, our bodies are pretty good at managing energy if we just trust them.

Many approaches to eating have a moralistic undertone. People who eat "healthy" or "clean" can consider themselves "good," while anyone who deviates from the rules is then "bad." This classification offers unlimited opportunities for mistakes, blame, shame, guilt, criticism, humiliation, condemnation, dissatisfaction, and self-loathing. Appealing energy-dense "bad" foods become associated with fear of loss of control, while nutrient-dense "good" foods become less appealing and boring. Tasty, likable foods become "guilty pleasures," often without regard to their actual nutrition, simply because they are enjoyable.

Meanwhile, the very word *healthy* has been hijacked for marketing purposes. The word appears on packaging and labeling everywhere because marketing people know that it increases sales. Sometimes it is used as a descriptor, such as "healthy snack," and sometimes it appears all alone. The last package of mushrooms I bought had the word "healthy" all by itself on the label. (I understand that there are poisonous mushrooms in the world, which are certainly unhealthy, but I would hope that they would not be found in a grocery store!) Guilt and shame are also woven into marketing. "Guilt-free" is used to describe cookies, while "sinfully rich" and "decadent" describe brownies and chocolate. An entire marketing campaign for ice cream is built around the phrase "guilt-free." A sign above a deli counter says, "Hummus you can feel good about." What kind of hummus should I not feel good about? Our insecurities about eating are used, once again, to separate us from our money. An interesting experiment is to go to the grocery store and deliberately try not to buy anything that is labeled in a way that promotes dieting mentality.

Shame and fear of shame are important dynamics in this discussion. Brene Brown, in her wonderful book *Women and Shame*, defines shame as "the intensely painful feeling or experience of believing we are flawed and therefore unworthy of acceptance and belonging."[2] Feeling flawed and unworthy because of a food choice seems pretty extreme, but it happens all the time, driven by a culture that has assigned moralistic values to the process of eating. Brown goes on to define *fundamentalism* as "any group espousing a belief system that holds itself so right and true that it discourages or even punishes questioning." When I read this, I immediately thought of a conversation I had with Jenny, a lovely lady with a graduate degree in theology, who came to see me for treatment of binge eating. She had been doing some online research on religious cults and said, "I suddenly realized that the description of the cult was eerily similar to the Weight Watchers meetings I used to attend!" One similarity was the idea that it is against the rules to question the rules.

Rigid, moralistic approaches to eating generally result in feelings of guilt and shame. When is it, in fact, appropriate to feel guilty about eating? I have not been able to think of an example. If I steal a coworker's lunch out of the break room refrigerator, I should feel guilty for stealing, not for eating. If I am an Orthodox Jew and eat something that is not kosher, I should feel guilty for violating my religious precepts, but not for eating. If I eat a big, juicy cheeseburger in front of a friend who is on a clear liquid diet because she is prepping for a medical procedure, I should feel guilty because that is just rude, not because I am eating.

A related and particularly troubling concept is *cheat days*. This involves following all the rules except when you do not follow them. On the surface, it seems to be a way around feelings of shame and guilt, but the label itself is associated with unworthiness. Cheating, by definition, involves dishonesty and unfairness. We do not get cheat days in algebra class, during tax season, or in our committed relationships. Eating what we want is not cheating; it is simply eating what we want.

A related concept is that of *treats*. When we define a food as a treat, we are giving it value beyond its nutrients. In the dieting culture, this is often identified as "anytime foods and sometimes foods" or "everyday vs. sometimes vs.

occasional foods." Once again, we have a hierarchy of foods based on their quality of being energy dense. What if we redefined treats based on a classification of monetary cost or effort? Lobster tails are a treat because we can only afford them occasionally. Twice-baked potatoes are a treat because they are labor intensive. Context matters, too. For example, my office is close to a grocery store that has a salad bar, where I often cross paths with a certain young man. One day, I commented, "We keep seeing each other here." He sighed and replied, "Yeah, I'm here a lot." I responded, "Yes, it's my weekly indulgence." He stopped moving, looked at me with surprise, and said, "Indulgence? Salad?" I replied, "Sure, paying these prices to get to choose exactly what I want, fresh and already cut up for me? I'm indulging myself!" I hope I helped him think a bit differently. People who focus on weight loss tend to think of salad as healthy/green light/anytime food, which then makes it less appealing, something they are *supposed* to eat instead of what they want. If all foods are good foods, salad can be delicious treat.

There are many ways that food can be valued, and all are dependent on context. Perhaps the most common example is when children are told that they can only have dessert if they finish their vegetables. This frames dessert as highly desirable and vegetables as a chore, or even punishment. When foods are considered a treat, they are being assigned an arbitrary value without much thought.

Consider the many other ways that food can be defined as having value. One is cost: lobster tails are expensive, which results in their being defined as a highly desirable food (at least for people who like lobster). By this measure, steak is more highly valued than hamburger, and salmon is more highly valued than chicken.

Another measure is availability. Some foods are only available at certain times, such as pumpkin pie at Thanksgiving. Girl Scout Cookies are marketed with this economy of scarcity idea. Because they are only available for a limited time each year, people get very excited about them and buy large quantities. If Girl Scout Cookies were available year-round, they would be much less special. Availability can also be geographic. If a favorite food item is only available in another city, then each time you visit that city, you are likely to seek out that food.

I had an interesting example of arbitrary food valuing several years ago at a conference that served a dessert buffet one evening. I generally travel with my own supply of chocolate, in case there is none available. Additionally, several of the tables in the exhibit hall had bowls of candy. When I arrived at the buffet, I saw a hot peach cobbler, which did not appeal to me; a lemon meringue pie; a carrot cake (personally, I have never understood the point of making a dessert out of a vegetable, but Underpants Rule); and a marble cake with that kind of icing that exists to look pretty rather than taste good, the only remotely chocolate item on the table. At the end of the table was a huge platter of fruit: plump grapes, juicy strawberries, and thin slices of melon fanned out in lovely designs. Now, it was March, so fruit was expensive in the stores. Additionally, someone else had invested all the labor into preparing and presenting the platter. I loaded up a plate with fruit and sat down at a table. A woman I had never seen before started in: "Oh, look, you're being so *good*, eating fruit, making the rest of us look *bad*, you're being so *good*!" I'd chosen the fruit because it was what appealed to me—it was expensive and labor intensive to prepare—but she assigned a completely different value to it. I finally went back and got a piece of cake just to get her to stop!

When food is both appealing and forbidden, it then gets labeled *bad* and becomes scary and unmanageable. This unfortunately common combination is a set up for a binge. When a food is labeled bad or otherwise prohibited, that idea is naturally followed with, "I can't ever have that again." The next time that particular food is encountered, it is extremely difficult to eat it in moderation because it is accompanied by the thought, "Once I finish this, I can never have it again." Bingeing is now a natural, obvious response. In contrast, labeling all foods as *good* foods allows a more considered intake because availability is not restricted. If you know you can have it now, or later, or next week, you will be satisfied more quickly and eat a reasonable amount. Obviously, some foods are only available at certain times, but that is not the same as being labeled as a bad food.

Additionally, the terms *junk food* and *processed food* are worth exploring. What exactly do they mean? Both terms are vague but carry a very negative connotation. Richard Wrangham, a primatologist, wrote a brilliant book called *Catching Fire: How Cooking Made Us Human.*[3] He makes the case that the physiological evolution of humans depended on the ability to cook food. He defines *processed* as anything that we do to food to make it edible and digestible, including cutting, mashing, cooking, soaking, or other preparation. If we simply chewed leaves, we would have to chew all day long to get enough energy to survive, leaving us no time for anything else. Yet, how often is processed food considered something to avoid, as not clean? I recently saw an article about a meal prep service that claimed "no processed foods," yet I am pretty sure it included things that had been cut up. Like *junk food*, it has become a poorly defined catchall term for "food I disapprove of."

If we try to avoid anything that is processed, where does that leave us with water? All of us consume processed water. There is a small river behind my house. I could walk down there and scoop up some unprocessed water, but it would not be safe to drink. Not everyone has access to safe drinking water, as it is only safe when properly processed. At the time of this writing, residents in Flint, Michigan, are still relying on bottled water, which is, of course, processed.

Trying to eat "healthy" or "clean" not only carries the potential for feelings of guilt and shame over small failures, but it can easily be carried to extremes.

The list of "acceptable" foods gets shorter and shorter, and life gets more and more constrained to avoid situations that might contain temptations to break the rules. Relationships and social lives suffer. Marilyn, a woman in her early sixties, was referred to me by her doctor, who was concerned about her weight loss. A self-described "fitness nut," she became obsessively focused on restrictive eating after dealing with a medical issue. By the time she came to me, her entire family was angry about the way her rules around food limited all their social interactions. We worked on healing those relationships as part of dealing with her eating disorder. She was making progress and had agreed to a family gathering at her grandchildren's favorite pizza parlor, but she backed out after hearing a local "health guru" on the radio deriding pizza as a terrible food. Her dieting rules and fears prevented her from enjoying an evening with her family. Her estrangement from them deepened when they stopped inviting her to social functions altogether.

Marilyn was suffering from orthorexia. Eating disorder treatment professionals have been identifying this pattern more and more often in recent years. While it is not yet an official diagnosis, orthorexia (*ortho* from the Greek for *upright* or *correct*) refers to a pattern of obsessive focus on eating right or clean or healthy that becomes so restrictive that it compromises nutritional status and limits life activities. Yet, these patterns are widely encouraged by "health gurus" of assorted backgrounds and training.

Once you start watching for these thought processes, they are everywhere. It is so common as to be unremarkable. At the end of a social function, how often do you hear, "Oh, please take this home with you, I can't have it in the house!" Why not? Because of the possibility of eating it? Consider what it would be like if, instead, the thought was, "I hope they leave me enough to have dessert for the next three days!" If all food is *good* food, it makes sense to save some for later or to eat it sparingly to make it last longer. The idea of food as dangerous is rarely questioned, but it is annoying and, ultimately, unhelpful. This was brought home to me recently when I went to a real estate agent's open house (because I love seeing the insides of old houses). The agent had baked chocolate chip cookies to fill the place with an appealing aroma, and a big plate of warm cookies sat next to the sign-in book. There was a covey of ladies in the next room who were talking among themselves about how they could not sign in because they could not get so close to the cookies. Their conversation quickly turned to a discussion of weight loss attempts, and I got a couple of glances as if they expected me to participate. I knew they did not want to hear what I had to say. For the record, the cookies were delicious, and I am sad that I seemed to be the only person able to enjoy them.

One of the effects of dieting mentality is a focus on *willpower* or *self-discipline* that always seems to play out in a negative way in relation to making "bad" food choices. If we remove the artificial valuing of foods as good or bad, we can make choices based on what we want and how we feel and save up our self-discipline for times when we need to clean house but would rather read a novel. If we are adequately nourished on a regular basis without any feelings of deprivation, we make better decisions about unexpected cookies based on how we feel in the moment.

These things seem inconsequential, but they are the background music of our lives; like a movie soundtrack, they influence our thoughts and feelings without always being noticeable. Make an effort to pay attention. Notice when conversation implies that eating behavior should be accompanied by avoidance, guilt, or shame. Listen to your own internal dialog about eating. If you feel guilty or label something a *bad food*, you are participating in dieting mentality. Observe and question the assumptions and implications. Consider how things might change if challenged.

Sometimes I hear people say, "Oh, I don't pay attention to any of that." My response is usually something along the lines of, "The quality of the water affects the fish that swim in it, whether the fish pays attention or not."

Our bodies need and deserve to be nourished in a dependable, predictable way. If the food we eat is tasty and appealing, there is no reason to feel shame, guilt, or unworthiness. All foods are good foods (unless they are spoiled or you are allergic to them). The ability to eat in moderation depends on permission to eat without self-reproach and blame.

When asked to name her guilty pleasures, the world-famous chef Julia Child is quoted as saying, "I don't have any guilt." What might that feel like?

Eat Enough

Chapter 3 discussed the concept of an internal locus of control. If you have been eating according to an external locus of control, counting on someone else to tell you what to eat, then relearning to eat according to your own signals takes time and practice. There are a number of ways to approach this. Please read the following suggestions through your own filter. Observe and be curious about your feelings while reading and also while implementing the ideas. If you notice anxiety, try and understand what that is about. If you feel guilt or shame, is that about breaking the dieting rules or is it about not being able to follow my suggestions? You have no obligation to do anything my way! Remember the Underpants Rule.

Hunger is an important signal, but it can be scary if you have been fighting against it for a long time. The longer a person has been undereating, the larger the hunger becomes. Restricting leads to bingeing. It is helpful to have a meal plan to ensure that you have enough to eat so that hunger does not become overwhelming. Eating according to your own internal signals is much easier when your body knows that it will be adequately and reliably nourished all the time.

Remember, a diet is focused on "Don't eat too much!" while a meal plan focuses on "Be sure to eat enough." To review, very general guidelines include eating at least three times a day; eating at least five servings of fruits and vegetables a day; eating at least five servings of complex carbohydrates (starches) a day; eating at least three servings of high-quality protein a day; and having a couple of servings of dairy every day. In addition to that, eat whatever you want. The "whatever you want" part may sound scary, but if you can follow the guidelines, your hunger will be manageable, and you will be more likely to eat a reasonable amount.

It is okay to start slowly. Eating at the same time every day helps the body to learn what to expect. If you regularly get too hungry before mealtime, add a snack or increase the amount in the previous meal. Be deliberate and mindful about the meals. Plan ahead so that you do not have to make decisions at the last minute. Pay attention to what you eat and how it tastes and feels. Notice how you feel afterward. Eat from plates or bowls rather than paper or cardboard whenever possible. Use real utensils.

Initially, it may be helpful to stick with foods that are not your particular favorites. Foods that you love are probably the ones you have been avoiding and/or bingeing on, so take some time to reestablish adequate nutrition before adding them. How can you make it safer when you do? This is easier with prepackaged foods. For example, if your main binge food is Oreos, when you are ready to try them again, buy a small package at the store, then go to a park and sit under the trees while you enjoy your Oreos. The different setting changes your perspective, and the small package size is a limited amount. If you want to binge, you have to go back to the store and buy more. You certainly can do that, but you also have time on the way to change your mind. This approach works with potato chips, ice cream, or any other packaged food. Reintroduce the item in circumstances that provide a reasonable limit. However, this is temporary; the goal is to become comfortable enough to keep foods on hand for whenever you feel like eating them. Think about what will help you feel safe while making the transition so that, eventually, you can feel relaxed about having larger quantities of food in the cabinets.

"Eat when you are hungry; stop when you are full" is easy to say but harder to do. Learning to assess your own hunger is challenging, so be forgiving of yourself if it takes time. Keep experimenting and paying attention. What, exactly, does hunger feel like to you? Sometimes it is a gnawing empty feeling; other times, it may be a mild discomfort. What is your hunger scale? Perhaps consider jotting down some ideas or descriptions to help you identify how hungry you are. Initially, at least, eat enough and often enough that you prevent feeling famished. How do you know that you are full? The goal is to be able to achieve satiety, a sense of being satisfied and adequately nourished, without being stuffed.

Sometimes we eat when we are not hungry, and that is fine, too. Perhaps we know that it will be awhile before we have a chance to eat again, and so we want to avoid feeling starved. While you are using a meal plan to restore your ability to eat intuitively, sometimes you will eat before you are aware of being hungry. Sometimes we eat just because it is there. "I need to eat" can be a thoughtful response to circumstances in the absence of physical hunger.

Remember to consider the message you give yourself about your own worth. Can you feel worthy enough to be selective? Can you, at least sometimes, have what you want exactly the way you want it? Be choosy without worrying what other people think. When planning and preparing food for a family, it is easy to focus on what everyone else wants. Conversely, when eating alone, it may feel like there is no point in going to any trouble. Fixing an appealing meal for oneself is a clear message about worth!

Eating should be a source of pleasure, not anxiety. Eating should be a delight, not a chore. Eating should be enjoyable. Meals that are prepared soulfully are more sustaining. Meals eaten with agreeable others are more satisfying. Meals that delight all the senses—taste, smell, touch, and vision— are more nourishing. Eat with love, not promiscuity. Eat with ritual, not haste. Can you learn to love how you feel after you eat?

Some of these suggestions may be easy to manage or already a part of what you do, but some may be more difficult. Be gentle with yourself. Each step you take moves you closer to being able to eat according to an internal locus of control, until it becomes easy. Remember the earlier discussion about setting small goals and paying attention to achieving them to build self-esteem. Try to do what feels manageable while continuing to take risks.

Breaking the Rules (or Go Ahead, Eat Your Entree with Your Salad Fork!)

Rules about food and eating range from formal etiquette, to cultural norms, to family traditions, to internalized dieting limitations and restrictions. Some of them, such as food safety rules, are obviously helpful. Others, such as prohibitions on eating birthday cake before the actual birthday, border on superstition. When food rules limit our ability to enjoy our lives, to be adequately nourished, or to feel good about ourselves, they need to be examined, understood, and then discarded. Food rules that result in feelings of anxiety, guilt, and shame are harmful, even when they are not focused on weight loss.

Slowing down and truly savoring food aids digestion and increases satisfaction. However, many customs teach us the opposite. Lois told me about how quickly her husband ate his meals; he was always finished before everyone else. Her husband grew up in a household where the last person done had to clean up the dishes. He continued to eat as if he were in a race! It was a habit that prevented him from fully enjoying his food. Vickie grew up with two brothers. She described a household where male appetites were considered more important than female needs; if her father or one of her brothers finished his piece of meat first, he would reach across the table with a fork, stab hers, and eat the rest. She learned to eat steak very quickly. Meanwhile, studies of school lunchrooms document that children eat more and throw away less when they have recess before lunch instead of after—because they are not rushing to get outside.

Consider what your food rules are, where they came from, and how to deliberately break them. (Obviously, this does not apply to food safety guidelines or actual medical limitations.) Let's start with that old standard, the Clean Plate Club. Eating everything on one's plate was and still is a standard expectation in many households. However, in some cultures, a clean plate is considered rude. This is sometimes referred to as "Leave a bite for Mr. Manners." If someone leaves an empty plate, then clearly the hostess did not provide enough to eat!

If we are eating according to internal cues that shift with our fullness, we need to be able to reevaluate how much we want. We may want a second helping, or we may leave some uneaten. No one can be expected to perfectly estimate how much they want to eat before they even start. If someone else has prepared the plate, as in a restaurant or banquet hall, then amounts are determined by an external locus of control, which provides an excellent opportunity to practice paying attention to internal feelings of fullness and satiety and stopping when comfortable, leaving some food uneaten. Make a deliberate effort to resign from the Clean Plate Club.

Consciously breaking the rules will likely raise anxiety, at least initially. What tools do you use in other parts of your life to manage anxiety? Focusing on your breath and mindfully relaxing muscle tension helps. Distractions, such as talking with another person, can be useful, with the understanding that the goal is to eventually be able to focus on the pleasure of eating without distraction. If the anxiety is intolerable, consider talking with a therapist or finding other resources to learn self-soothing tools. Go slowly enough to be successful while making some progress.

Lydia grew up with the household rules that no one could eat dinner before dad got home and eating could only happen at the dining room table. As her father was an unpredictable alcoholic, this often resulted in overcooked meals, ravenously hungry children, and exceptionally unpleasant dinnertime experiences. As an adult, her anxiety about eating affected her health to the point that her physician sent her to see me. In addition to talking about her history, I encouraged her to experiment with intentionally breaking the rules by eating alone, at different times, and in different rooms in her house. We talked about and practiced ways for her to manage the anxiety that she felt when she broke the rules. Her rules were not about weight loss, but they were still debilitating.

Many dieting rules focus on the efforts to eat less to lose weight, and yet we know that the body will adapt metabolically and that restriction generally leads to overeating. Still, the rules can be difficult to identify and change. Let's look at some.

Drink a glass of iced water before a meal. This is supposed to fill up the stomach and reduce the amount of food eaten while requiring more calories to warm the water. Hunger will return sooner. The body cannot be fooled, at least not for long. A related rule tries to fool the stomach by keeping it filled with water all day long, as in "Keep a glass of water on your desk." Drinking enough water is a good plan because water is essential for life, not because it tricks you into eating less.

Use a smaller plate. If the plate looks full, you will feel more full with less food. Maybe, but you will get hungry again sooner.

Fill up on low-calorie, low-carb vegetables. You may get full, but you will not be satisfied. This may also interfere with your ability to enjoy vegetables.

Chew gum. Again, this is tricking your mouth into being happy with no intake. Notice how many dieting rules and suggestions are focused on tricking the body into thinking that it is full when it is not.

Weigh yourself every day. Daily weighing increases anxiety, guilt, and obsessional worry. It does not provide any helpful information. If the number goes up, the response is, "Oh, no, I have to redouble my efforts to lose weight." If the number stays the same, the response is, "Oh, no, I have to redouble my efforts to lose weight." If the number goes down, the response is, "Oh, great! Now I have to redouble my efforts to lose weight." The number on the scale does not measure your worth, your health, or your success in meeting your goals. Daily weighing provides a false sense of being in control. Many people initially feel anxious about not knowing their weight but find that it leads to less distress.

Obviously, there are some medical exceptions to this advice. People who have congestive heart failure need to weigh every day. On the other hand, treatment for eating disorders, especially anorexia nervosa, usually involves *blind weights*, in which the individuals are weighed with their backs to the scale by a therapist, dietician, or nurse so that they know that their weight is being monitored without having to worry about it themselves.

Write down everything you eat, or keep a food journal. Again, this increases anxiety about eating and about remembering to write it down. Just like daily weighing, it encourages an external locus of control instead of paying attention to internal hunger cues. It also has the potential to increase dishonesty.

Eat more fiber. This is supposed to increase feelings of fullness, but the body knows when it does not get enough to eat. Healthwise, many people could benefit from eating more fiber because it makes their digestive systems work better, not because it creates a false sense of fullness.

Portion control: Measure out all servings. Because someone else knows better than you do about how much you want. Measuring is an external locus of control that increases anxiety and decreases body trust.

Shop from a list, only buy what is on it, and pay cash. This is supposed to reduce impulse food buying, but having a good overall relationship with food is a better way to decrease impulsive eating decisions.

Read labels. Again, this is an external locus of control. At some point, when you are more comfortable in your relationship with food, it may be interesting to read the labels for general information (there may not be as much protein in that protein bar as you thought), but, initially, it may lead you to decisions that are not about what you really want.

Serve from the cooking utensils. Supposedly, having serving dishes on the table leads to eating more than you "should." If you are still hungry, or it is simply more delicious than you thought, have seconds. Having permission to take more is part of learning to make choices based on an internal locus of control. Also, if we are trying to make mealtime a delightful social affair, serving up from a pot on the stove kind of defeats the purpose.

Wear a tight belt. Because feeling uncomfortable all day long will motivate you to be meaner to your body by eating less than you need. How is this possibly a good idea?

Throw out your "fat" clothes. Years ago, at an eating disorder conference, I heard an idea about how the women's clothing industry benefits from weight cycling by selling the new wardrobe that is often the reward for weight loss. Then the stores sell more clothes, to replace the "fat" clothes that were thrown out, when the weight is inevitably regained. The industry would lose money if we all stayed the same size.

Don't eat when you are not hungry. This commandment is common and very detrimental. First of all, how do you define *hunger*? Does your stomach have to rumble? Do you have to be lightheaded? Are you hungry enough to justify eating without shame? Second, it negates life experience and context. Sometimes we eat before we are hungry because we know it will be awhile before we can eat again. Sometimes we eat because a yummy opportunity presents itself. We can trust our bodies to accommodate.

Exercise to justify or make up for food intake. Again, this is very common but not benign. Whether it sounds like "I can eat this because I worked out" or "I will have to work out if I eat this," it is an opportunity to make a mistake that is followed by shame. Eating is about providing our bodies with nutrition. Exercise is about feeling good moving our bodies. Sitting still requires food, too. Eating and exercise do not cancel each other out; they are completely separate activities with different purposes.

Don't eat after (something) o'clock. This is related to equating intake with exercise by saying that we do not need energy if we are going to be sleeping, even though the basal metabolic rate (BMR) accounts for much of our energy needs. Your body still needs energy when it is at rest. If certain foods cause you to have gastric reflux or bad dreams, paying attention to your own responses can guide your decisions. The idea that anything you eat before bed turns into fat is bunk.

Don't drive down the street where your favorite bakery is located. If you are paying that much attention, you have probably been thinking about your favorite bakery item all day, so avoiding it may lead to overeating something else in compensation. Enjoy the doughnut or cupcake and get on with your life.

When eating salad, have the dressing on the side, then dip your fork into it before spearing the vegetables. This is supposed to limit or eliminate calories. What it actually does is limit or eliminate pleasure and enjoyment. Meanwhile, it is perfectly fine to order the dressing on the side in a restaurant so that you can have exactly the amount that you consider the most enjoyable instead of what the person in the kitchen thinks is the right amount.

Eat breakfast every day. Okay, this is actually a good idea. It is a way to remind yourself that you deserve to be nourished and satisfied.

Wherever you find ideas like those above, whether they are described as rules, guidelines, or "secrets to success," they are based on using an external locus of control to trick your body into getting by with less nutrition than it needs. They may be framed as healthy or good self-care, but they ultimately undermine your faith in your body's wisdom. Following them leads to hunger, deprivation, weight cycling, lower self-worth, and, possibly, binge eating.

Moderation is not possible if your body expects deprivation. Pay attention to your own "rules" and question how they promote deprivation. Consider how you can challenge and change them.

Dieting rules, like many sets of rules, encourage an all-or-nothing mindset. Once one rule is broken, they might as well all be broken. Systems based on an external locus of control promote the extremes of compliance versus defiance. Trying to perfectly follow impossible requirements often leads to an attitude of, "Oh yeah? You can't tell me what to do! Just watch me!" In some circumstances, that defiance and oppositionality is helpful in getting out of a bad situation or surviving while protecting a sense of identity when the situation cannot be escaped. If alternating between compliance and defiance with dieting rules is a habit for you, giving up the rules may be disorienting at first.

One of the purposes of rules is that they make decision making easier. Defying the rules may lead to anxiety and a fear of losing control. Be kind with yourself; go slowly if you need to, but notice how the rules limit your autonomy. Keep challenging them. If your feelings are too much to manage, consider finding a therapist who understands the Health At Every Size approach and make an appointment.

Accept No Substitutions (or Cherry Coke Is Not a Fruit)

> Abby opened the fridge and pulled out the carrots and a green pepper. She eyed the shelf with the salad dressing. Blue cheese, Thousand Island, and fat-free ranch. The fat-free ranch was for her. It tasted like garlicky glue with artificial sweetener stirred in. She wondered if she could sneak some Thousand Island on her salad when no one was looking.[4]

This quote is from the delightful children's book *The Second Life of Abigail Walker*. It is about a girl who finds a way to be her true self despite parents who want her to lose weight. It captures the problem with "substitute" food, which is unappealing and unsatisfying. It also speaks to how an external locus of control can lead to cheating and secretive eating.

Many enjoyable foods can lose their appeal if they are regularly substituted for something else in an attempt to decrease energy intake and are based on a vague similarity. One example is spaghetti squash, the flesh of which forms long strands that are somewhat similar in shape to pasta. It does not taste like pasta, and it does not have the same texture as pasta. But dieting recipes encourage the use of spaghetti squash because it is somehow better than pasta. Spaghetti squash is a delicious vegetable (to be fair, I have never met a squash I did not like), but it is not pasta. Trying to pretend that the foods are interchangeable will lead to disappointment. Regular pasta has a place in a meal plan because it contains energy and vitamins; also, it is delicious.

A similar example is the use of cauliflower in place of potatoes. What do cauliflower and potatoes have in common? They are both white. In terms of flavor and texture, they are very different. Yet, some dieting tips recommend substituting mashed cauliflower for mashed potatoes.

Historically, most human cuisines have a basic starchy food as their foundation, whether it is pasta, bread, potatoes, rice, or corn. These foods provide considerable energy, which is a necessary part of nutrition. They may provide the base of a dish, functioning to hold up a sauce made from other foods. Pasta holds up marinara or pesto. Mashed potatoes hold up gravy. The relatively neutral taste and texture allow the more complicated topping to be appreciated. The taste of cauliflower does not blend well with the taste of gravy, and ditto for mashed turnips. Pesto on spaghetti squash does not sound very appealing either.

Portobello mushrooms may have the same shape as a hamburger, but they do not have the same flavor, texture, or nutritional value. Ground turkey does not taste the same as ground beef. Prune puree may work instead of butter when baking, but the flavor will be different. Fruit is not "nature's candy." It is fruit, which is yummy. Candy is yummy, too. Candy has a place in a meal plan, as does fruit. They should not be substituted for each other.

Marketing experts know that they can use dieting mentality to sell products. The food itself may be the same, but the label changes. For example, when I was an undergraduate taking foods and nutrition classes (decades ago), one of the topics we studied was cheese. We learned about the process of making cheese and what the differences were in various types. We learned that cream cheese was made from cream and Neufchâtel cheese was almost the same thing but made from milk, which meant it was cheaper. The thrifty housewife could substitute it for cream cheese in most recipes. Now, Neufchâtel cheese is labeled "low-fat cream cheese" and costs the same. Foods that are labeled "low in sugar" or "low-fat" may be the same as they have always been, but they sell better when they are marketed to appeal to restrictive eaters.

When we try to substitute a lower calorie food for what we really want, we are unlikely to be satisfied with the outcome. However, letting go of the dieting mentality opens up the possibility of enjoying foods for what they are. Some folks find portobello mushrooms to be delicious as mushrooms. Ground turkey may taste better than ground beef for some recipes. If you really like the taste of turkey (as I do), you may find that you like turkey sausage better than traditional simply because of the flavor, not because of the "healthier" nutritional content. Experiment and see what you like. You may be surprised.

For instance, what kind of salad dressing do you like, really like, regardless of the calorie content? I have always thought that commercial low-fat and fat-free dressings are nasty and, fortunately, avoidable. Several years ago, I went to the trouble of making myself a fresh salad only to discover that the bottle of my favorite ranch dressing was almost empty. I poured a little malt vinegar into the bottle and shook it up to get the last bits. It was delicious! I decided that was how I wanted to eat my salad always. It was much later before it occurred to me that I had essentially invented my own version of "lite" dressing. I have experimented with other kinds of vinegar, but malt is my favorite. Once you let go of the dieting mentality, you may be pleasantly surprised at what you really like or do not like.

Can you have exactly what you want, exactly the way you want it, at least some of the time? Can you spend some time figuring out what that means? Many people have difficulty in asking for what they want, especially if they have a long history of feeling undeserving or unworthy. Elsa told me about a coffee dilemma. Her one "indulgence" was going to a drive-through window each morning on her way to work to get a cup of coffee. She actually liked it with three creams and four sugars, but she asked for less so that the person taking her order did not have to go to a second screen on the computer. She had difficulty asking for what she wanted in other aspects of her life as well. Learning to ask for her coffee exactly the way she wanted and expecting the service she was paying for was a step in becoming more assertive elsewhere in her life. What are you settling for when you deserve better?

Similarly, Angela loved watermelon, but she never bought it for herself because no one else in her family liked it. If she could not eat a whole watermelon by herself, then buying one was "wasteful," and buying the jars of preprepared watermelon was too expensive. Eating watermelon became a way for her to embrace the idea that she was worthy and deserving.

Savor your food. Enjoyment is not dangerous; food is not the enemy. When possible, get what you want, the way you want it, then take pleasure in eating. One of the fallacies about food and weight is that "enjoying food too much" is a problem. In fact, people who truly take delight in what they eat tend to be satisfied with less because they are paying attention to taste and sensation. Chronic deprivation leads to a feeling of being insatiable, but this feeling fades with adequate nutrition. Let yourself enjoy!

Notice any patterns of eating secretly or defiantly. Betty was a plump middle-aged woman whose naturally slender husband nagged at her about her weight and monitored her food intake at home. When she had to make a long car trip by herself, she stopped multiple times on the way to get french fries, which she gobbled in privacy while driving. She was careful to clean out the car before going home again. While it is understandable that she wanted to avoid criticism from her judgmental husband, it is sad that she could not allow herself to enjoy her fries without distraction. If you notice secrecy or defiance in some aspect of your eating, can you be mindful of that and find a safe way to be more open and direct?

Food and Morality

How do we decide who is a good person? How do we judge good behavior? In recent years, what we eat and how much we weigh have taken on a value that goes far beyond health and appearance. Susan Greenhalgh's outstanding book *Fat-Talk Nation* addresses the societal imperative to be a "good biocitizen," which requires being or becoming thin, then badgering everyone else into becoming thin. She contends that the focus on fatness is not about health; it is about morality.[5]

In some ways, the concept of *clean eating* is a natural result of defining morality based on body size. There is no clear definition of what clean eating is, but everything that is not clean eating is, by definition, *dirty eating*. Who would want to eat dirty? Deciding to eat clean is a slippery slope into guilt and shame. The more rules there are, the more opportunities there are to get it wrong.

Furthermore, many of the moralistic recommendations also ignore social inequities. It might be great to eat locally sourced, organically grown, minimally processed foods, but doing so requires a certain amount of time, money, and access. It is much easier to be a good biocitizen if you are rich. When you see articles or suggestions about how people *should* eat, see if you can evaluate them in terms of moral values and assumptions that leave out a large part of the population or promote shame. Can you distance yourself from the guilt and shame they promote? (I will explore this topic in more detail in chapter 7.)

Everyone deserves to eat enough, to eat on a regular basis, and to eat food that is tasty and enjoyable and that meets their nutritional needs. Everyone is worthy of living a comfortable life, free from unnecessary guilt and shame.

As Anthony Warner says, "A healthy diet is one of joy, not one of rejection and denial. If you want to eat for health, you should have nothing to do with the creation of arbitrary, senseless rules and should never feel the lightest guilt over an occasional indulgence."[6]

CHAPTER FIVE

Healing the Self-Hate Injuries, Reclaiming Body Joy

Because, um, excuse me, this body you're in? Yeah, I think that's yours. You're the only one who can provide it with the things that help it work better and feel better, and help you work better and feel better and think better with regard to your body and your self.

—Hanne Blank, *The Unapologetic Fat Girl's Guide to Exercise and Other Incendiary Acts*[1]

Body dissatisfaction and self-hatred are so common in our culture that they have become unremarkable. It does not have to be that way. In many ways, body loathing is a habit that we can change. We only get one body in this lifetime, and we all deserve to feel good in the bodies we have. The weight loss industry promotes the idea that our bodies have to change before we can feel good about ourselves, but no amount of change is ever enough. The alternative is to stop buying into that message and to find ways to appreciate the body you have right now, the way it is today.

Everyone has moments of not liking their body for various reasons, but those moments should be fleeting. Our bodies do wonderful things for us all the time, all day long. As you read this, your heart is circulating your blood, your lungs are oxygenating that blood, and your brain is taking nutrients from that blood to enable you to process the information on the page. And your body does all of this without any conscious intention on your part. Isn't that amazing?

Your body deserves your appreciation, and you deserve to live in your body with joy and pleasure.

Life is filled with opportunities to internalize negative messages about our bodies. These messages come from our parents, our friends, our gym teachers, from the media, and other sources: "Your face is spotty," "Your teeth are crooked," "Your hair is stringy," or "You would be so pretty if you lost some weight."

Spend some time listening to your own internal dialog for the body messages that make you feel bad about yourself. Perhaps write them down and find a neutral phrase to substitute instead. The new phrase does not have to be glowingly wonderful (you would not believe it anyway), just different. You do not need to say, "My teeth are beautiful," but rather, "My teeth do a good job of chewing the food I need to be nourished."

When you listen to the thoughts in your head, consider what they would sound like if you said them out loud to someone else. A woman I met at a workshop shared that when she verbalized her self-shaming thoughts, her husband would say, "I don't like hearing you talk about my best friend that way." Can you be your own best friend? If not, can you think of someone who can say that to you, even if only in your imagination?

Again, there is a value that has been promoted in many ways that shaming can change behavior. We have come to believe that the best way to improve ourselves is by self-shaming, yet research clearly shows that those who feel good about themselves have better health behaviors and better physical and mental health.[2] Self-acceptance and self-appreciation are antidotes to self-shame.

Learning to accept and appreciate our bodies is challenging in a culture where some people make money from stealing our self-esteem so that they can sell it back to us at a profit. We may not be able to change the culture, but we can change how we respond to it. Can you develop a habit of questioning the messages that you hear, not only from the media but from the people around you? Notice the comments that promote body dissatisfaction and challenge them in your mind. Maybe someday you can challenge them out loud.

Lisa came to see me because of her disordered eating, which she had kept secret for years. She was, conventionally, very attractive but struggled with a negative body image. While we were discussing strategies for feeling more comfortable in a swimsuit during a family vacation, she shared her concerns about talking with her mother, who often made disparaging comments about other people's bodies. Lisa was, understandably, unwilling to discuss her own body dissatisfaction with her mother, so we took a suggestion from Ragen Chastain[3] and planned a response: "I wish we could all live in a society that valued all bodies, regardless of their size." This prepared answer gave Lisa the courage she needed to wear her swimsuit at the resort.

Self-care is a good start for changing your sense of body satisfaction. Getting enough sleep; enough tasty, nutritious food; and enough joyful movement are all steps toward appreciating your body, exactly as it is. Other pleasurable experiences, such as bubble baths, massages, or comfortable clothes, also contribute to a sense of well-being.

An often overlooked resource that we can access any time is our breath. Breathing is usually automatic, but it can also manage anxiety and discomfort while helping us stay centered and grounded. We frequently hear, "Take a deep breath! Just take a deep breath!" but we rarely talk about what that actually means. I regularly talk with my clients about using breath to deal with anger and anxiety, and I ask them to show me a deep breath. Almost always, they breathe with a noticeable up-and-down movement of the chest and no movement below that. I then instruct them to place a hand on the chest and a hand on the belly, below the navel, and to try to keep the hand on the chest still while pushing out the hand on the belly. Most people have difficulty with this, unless they sing, play a wind instrument, or practice yoga. On occasion, I have had women say, "I can't do that! I can't let my stomach stick out like that!" The cultural compulsion to "Suck in your gut!" keeps us from breathing the way we should and contributes to anxiety.

One good way to practice this is to find a big book, lie down on your back, and place the book low on your belly. Focus on moving the book up and down with your breath to get the feel of it. This is actually an exercise used by voice teachers. When you think you have it, practice breathing while sitting up, walking around, and doing other movements (do not hyperventilate). Take a few moments each day to practice so it is easy to remember when you need it. This kind of breathing can help manage uncomfortable feelings, whether they are anxiety about eating, uncertainty about your body, or anger that you are only now noticing because you are no longer distracting yourself with dieting.

Mind-Body Split

To heal someone, you need to change their way of thinking, if only for a moment.

—C. E. Murphy, from *Urban Shaman*[4]

Many of us feel like we live our lives in our heads, while our bodies are something that needs to be "managed." How do we heal that mind-body split? In addition to noticing and changing our thinking, we can also focus on new ways to inhabit and experience our bodies. We can do this sitting still, but it is more effective to do it while we are moving.

Now we come to another of those words laden with emotion and judgment: exercise. All too commonly, *exercise* means a way to lose weight, a punishment for being too fat, or a way to make up for eating. It becomes penance for the sin of having an unmanageable body. In reality, we all move, one way or another. Can we reclaim movement as something joyful, as a better way to inhabit our bodies? (I am going to use the "E-word"; feel free to substitute other words, such as *activity* or *movement*, if it helps you feel more comfortable.)

It might be worthwhile to sit for a few minutes and observe your feelings about exercise. It is not uncommon for those who struggle with body and weight issues to internalize some very negative attitudes about physical activity. Ask yourself, "Do I equate movement with eating as a way to burn off calories? Do I scold myself for eating by forcing myself to exercise? Do I consider exercise contrition for the sin of weighing too much? Where and when did I learn these ideas?" These and similar questions may help you clarify your thinking. If considering them is too uncomfortable to tolerate, it might be useful to find a Health At Every Size–informed therapist to help you.

Physical activity is another way that we give ourselves a message about what we think we are worth. If we hate what we are doing, if we feel awful, either physically or mentally, we are giving ourselves a clear message. If we find something to do that gives us joy and pleasure, that allows us to appreciate our extraordinary bodies; that is a different message. Our internal narrative matters, too. If our thoughts focus on changing our unacceptable bodies, we are not going to feel the same way as if we remind ourselves that we are taking good care of ourselves.

Exercise can be redefined as something we do for self-care, another way to love and value ourselves in the bodies that we have. Keep in mind that exercise and eating are two completely different activities, with different purposes and outcomes. We eat to nourish ourselves, to enjoy food, and to socialize. We exercise for joy and pleasure and because we feel better when we do. Be aware of any thoughts that equate exercise with food, as in, "I need to go work out because I had seconds at lunch" or "I can eat this because I ran two miles this morning." You eat because you eat. You move because you move. Both activities count as self-care. They do not cancel each other out.

Exercise promotes a feeling of competence and security in our own bodies. Movement is a way to reconnect with our wonderful selves and be aware of our own physical power. When we fully inhabit our bodies, we can fully inhabit our own lives. To quote Paul Linden, "A good body technology is worth twice its weight in philosophy."[5]

The physical benefits of exercise are widely known: improved blood pressure, better cardiac health, less insulin resistance, and lower cholesterol, among others. Exercise also has benefits for emotional and mental health. It raises the serotonin (the "feel good" hormone) levels in the brain, lowers stress hormones in the bloodstream, improves memory and learning, and improves sleep. It does all this independent of weight loss.

Yet, how often do people measure exercise success by the numbers on the scale? If someone decides to "get healthy" by working out and losing weight, that person will get discouraged if the numbers on the scale do not go down quickly enough (or at all) and probably give up. This takes us back to goal setting. Behavioral goals for exercise might include the following:

- I will walk for 15 minutes three times a week.
- I will take the stairs instead of the elevator when I come back to my office from lunch.
- I will go to yoga class twice a week.

Subjective measures of success include the following:

- I will be able to walk up a flight of stairs without being out of breath.
- I will be able to get up and down off the floor while playing with my children.
- I will pay attention to whether I focus better at work.
- I will pay attention to how well I sleep.

Physical measures such as blood pressure, cholesterol, and A1C (a measure of how well your body uses insulin over time) are more difficult to evaluate because measuring them requires equipment or blood tests; changes can be small and incremental over time, but they are important, too. All of these improvements are overlooked when success is measured by the numbers on the scale.

I'm often asked, "What is the best kind of exercise to do?" My answer is always, "It's the one you will continue doing." There is no one form of physical activity that is right for everyone. If you hate it, it is definitely the wrong one. How much exercise is the right amount? Again, that depends. If you have been completely sedentary, then walking for 10 minutes at a time, two or three times a week, may be a good place to start. If that is too much, try walking the length of your household hallway a couple of times a day. If you are unable to walk, perhaps try some upper body movement with or without small hand weights for 10 minutes at a time, three times a week.

If you are already active, think about the optimal amount and type of exercise for you. Research information about this is variable and conflicting, but the most common recommendation seems to be that 150 minutes a week results in measurable general health benefits; more than that may not produce much additional advantage. Of course, anyone who is training for something specific, like a marathon or a sport, will see improvement in certain abilities with more time than that, but if your focus is to feel better and inhabit your body more lovingly, then set your goals accordingly. Moving in a way that raises your heart rate for 30 minutes five times a week, or 50 minutes three times a week, or 22 minutes a day is enough to achieve health goals. It is not necessary to work out at the gym for two hours every day (unless you want to, because Underpants Rule).

Much of what we see in the media about exercise focuses on appearance, even though appearance is very difficult to change. When we think about function instead, we bring a new awareness to how we feel and how we experience our bodies. "Time to shape up for swimsuit season!" may sell weight loss products, but focusing on how well your body works is more sustainable. Goals such as stamina, flexibility, and balance will make you feel better without necessarily putting your money into someone else's pocket. Exercise should help you feel powerful, not insecure.

What kind of movement gives you joy? What might you like to try? What variables do you need to consider? If the goal is to learn to inhabit your body more fully with pleasure and satisfaction, you may need to rethink your ideas about movement. Can you use an internal locus of control to think about what you enjoy? The same way you ask yourself, "What am I hungry for right now?" you can ask yourself, "How does my body want to move right now?" It may not always be possible to move that way, but asking the question may provide more information.

"Saying 'I'm not flexible so I can't do yoga' is like saying 'I'm hungry so I can't eat that sandwich'" (Megan, my yoga teacher, comment on Facebook).

When I talk with people about exercise classes, I often hear, "I can't do yoga/Pilates/Zumba/kickboxing. I'm not any good at it." Everyone starts as a beginner; it is rare for someone to be good at something the first time they try. You do not go to Wimbledon to learn to play tennis!

Sometimes it is helpful to make a deliberate decision to do something you are not good at as a way to learn to tolerate imperfection. You also do not have to be good at something to enjoy it. As a young adult, I took several different types of dance classes. I was adequate at some of them, but my favorite was Dunham Technique (a type of modern dance that incorporates African and Haitian movements). I was perfectly dreadful at it, but I loved the way I felt in my body when I did it. Some years later, I wandered into a Tae Kwon Do class (because my children were taking it and loved it). I thought I knew how to feel powerful in my body, but suddenly I realized, "Oh! This is *different!*" I spent the next several years being not very good at martial arts. Now I take an advanced yoga class where I just adapt the poses rather than struggle to keep up with the skinny twisty bendy girls (at least one of whom is literally one-third my age) because I love it and leave with good body thoughts.

Good body thoughts and bad body thoughts is a concept that does not get nearly enough attention in the fitness world. Bad body thoughts are often the default, but they shouldn't be. Our bodies are amazing, and we deserve to feel good about them. When you engage in a physical activity, pay attention to your thoughts. If you have bad body thoughts, is it because that is your habit, or is it because of the activity itself? Especially in class settings or group activities, if the leader behaves or talks in a way that promotes bad body thoughts, evaluate that carefully. It may be that you need to try again with a different instructor before perhaps deciding to change activities altogether. If bad body thoughts are a habit, experiment with identifying, challenging, and changing them. Instead of "I was awful at that," substitute "That was fun and I might have been marginally better than last time!"

What to Do?

There are many factors to consider when thinking about physical activity, whether you are just starting out or are already active but want to change it up. What do you enjoy? Again, the prevailing attitude is that activity only counts if it leads to weight loss, so you may not have thought much about what you enjoy. Sometimes the information you have used to make the decisions may not even be accurate. Jill, a large young woman who came to see me about relationship issues, happened to tell me that she loved swimming but gave it up. Someone told her that swimming did not lead to weight loss because swimmers do not sweat. First of all, sweating and weight loss are not the same thing. Second, how would you know whether someone is sweating if they are in a pool of water? I encouraged her to engage in the activity she loved because she loved it. What do you love? What kind of movement makes you feel joyous?

Of course, there are practical considerations. You might love surfing but live in Indiana or Wyoming. You might love playing soccer but cannot afford the expenses of a traveling team. You might love running but your knees have a different opinion. Within the very real limits of your life, what is possible? Do you like being with other people or do you prefer working out alone? Do you enjoy classes that happen on a schedule or does it work better for you to be on your own timetable? Do you prefer fast-paced action or something more contemplative? Do your finances allow for club memberships and special clothing or do you need to be frugal? Do you want to make new friends or be left alone?

Consider different options. Hula-Hooping can be done alone or in groups and requires little financial outlay. It is good for balance and literally helps you feel more centered. Dance classes can enhance a sense of creativity. Martial arts can improve self-confidence. Yoga may lead to improved resilience to stress (plus, no shoes!). What sounds like fun to you? Libraries and community centers often offer classes that are low cost or free.

If you decide to try a class of some sort, there are additional considerations beyond the type of activity. Do you want the experience to also expand your social life? I have taken classes where no one ever spoke to each other, and I have taken classes where the members got together for potluck dinners on the weekend. The teaching style of the instructor matters, too. It is okay to choose which class to attend based on the instructor, especially in big dance, yoga, or martial arts studios with extensive schedules. Personally, I make it a practice to never take a class with an instructor who promotes any kind of diet mentality. I have been known to walk out of class after a comment like, "Let's burn off some of those holiday calories!"

One of the advantages of taking a class is the opportunity to stop thinking and deciding for an hour, or however long the class lasts. For those of us with busy days and many demands on our time, it is refreshing to let someone else be in charge for a bit. Whether it is dance, yoga, or judo, the instructor is the one who decides what to do next, how long to do it, and when to move on. This allows our brains to take a minivacation in a way that is difficult to achieve in a solo practice.

Many people enjoy working out at a gym, which usually requires a membership of some sort. Obvious considerations for gym membership include cost, geographic availability, and hours of operation. Additionally, think about how comfortable the atmosphere feels before agreeing to give anyone your money. Does the clientele include people of a variety of ages, body sizes, and capabilities, or is it mostly young, bodybuilder types? Are they dressed in assorted workout clothes or fitted designer togs? Are there charts on the walls promoting weight loss or low body fat percentages? If there are "inspirational" posters, do you actually find them inspiring? Do you see anything that promotes body shame? Overall, does the place encourage good body thoughts or bad body thoughts for you?

Most gym memberships will include a free orientation session with a trainer to review the safe use of the equipment, plus the option of paying for additional sessions. Keep in mind that personal trainers are exposed to the same inaccurate, toxic information about weight as the rest of the culture, and they may or may not buy into it. A good trainer will ask you about your own goals and help you work toward improved strength, stamina, balance, or whatever your goals may be. If a trainer tries to push his or her own beliefs about weight loss, find a new trainer. If the trainer ignores your own capabilities and pushes you too much, speak up!

Janet, who originally came to see me about family problems, told me about a trainer she had worked with at a local gym. He seemed to take it as a challenge to work her to her maximum, and she did not want to disappoint him. She told me that after each session, she would rush to the ladies locker room, vomit repeatedly, and then lie on the floor in a cold sweat for a half hour before being able to shower. Shortly after that, she stopped going to the gym altogether, relinquishing any benefit she could have had from a more reasonable workout because of her increased sense of shame.

A common reason for not exercising is "I don't have time." Certainly, most of us have more to do than we have time to do it in, but we are more effective in our daily lives if we take the time to take care of ourselves. Part of the benefit of exercise is carving out a chunk of time for ourselves and making our own needs a priority. It is about saying, "You all are just going to have to manage without me for 30 minutes because I'm going for a walk," or perhaps, "Your question is going to have to wait until tomorrow because I'm on my way to yoga." We need to take some time to simply focus on our own well-being, even if we spend the time sitting on a park bench. Part of the benefit comes from saying, "I'm worth it."

Some people find fitness trackers to be helpful and motivating, but, again, evaluate the self-care benefits for yourself. Chasing young grandchildren is certainly satisfying and may rack up an impressive number of steps on your phone, but there is a different benefit involved in walking outside, letting your mind wander, feeling the breeze on your face, and having no responsibilities for a few minutes. If you use a fitness tracker, does it motivate you or give you another excuse to not take time for yourself? Someone recently told me about overhearing, "I forgot to wear my tracker today, so my steps don't count." How does that factor into the message you give yourself about your own worth?

> "'Discipline'?" Mieka exclaimed. "What a frightful word! *Discipline* is forcing yourself to do what you don't want to do. Doesn't take any *discipline* to be doing what you love!"[6]

Whatever you decide to do, make it pleasurable enough to continue. Can you find something you enjoy? Can you find a way to make what you are already doing more enjoyable? You deserve to have a good experience at the gym, the class, the park, or wherever you choose to be physically active. Do not put up with bad experiences; complain or go somewhere else. You deserve to enjoy being active in your body.

For more ideas and information, I highly recommend Hanne Blank's excellent book *The Unapologetic Fat Girl's Guide to Exercise and Other Incendiary Acts*[7] as well as Jeanette DePatie's *The Fat Chick Works Out! (Fitness That's Fun and Feasible for Folks of All Ages, Sizes, Shapes and Abilities)*.[8] (To be clear, Dr. Blank identifies as the Unapologetic Fat Girl, and Ms. DePatie identifies as the Fat Chick; you are not required to identify as either to benefit from the books.)

I would like to share my own philosophy about exercise: "No pain—great!"

CHAPTER SIX

Dealing with the World: Weight Stigma, Part 1

You have stuck with me this far, and you are still reading! I hope you have learned some things you did not know before about the science of weight and health and about ways to nourish and move your body to improve your self-esteem and your quality of life. Hopefully, you are already putting some of these ideas into practice in your everyday routines.

Unfortunately, sooner or later, you have to go back out into a world that does not agree. Most of the rest of the world still buys into the myths that we have been debunking, and they do not want to hear your new truth. What do you do?

Weight stigma is an uncomfortable topic, but it is an important one to understand. It is so deeply woven into the fabric of our culture as to be invisible. It can be institutional or personal, obvious or covert, clear or subtle.

Weight stigma can be thought of as a type of bullying. It is important to remember that, with bullying, the behavior of the bully is the problem. Bullying cannot be defeated by making the victim more acceptable to the bully. Weight stigma cannot be solved by trying to make your body more acceptable to those who still believe that fat people should be shamed into being smaller.

The world is a difficult place for fat people. They make less money, are less likely to be promoted, and are portrayed in the media in ways that are derogatory and disparaging. They are bullied and mistreated in schools, on the street, in doctors' offices and even in their own homes. Discrimination against fat people in our culture is very real. And they are told it is their own fault.

The concept of weight stigma is complicated and multifaceted. It is grounded in the faulty assumptions that weight is under an individual's control and that shame is a useful motivating tool. It is very much promoted by the $64 billion a year weight loss industry. There is money to be made by making people feel shame about their bodies. It is so much a part of our culture that most people do not even notice, which makes it immeasurably more damaging. The reality is that being fat in the world is crappy, which makes it something to be avoided. However, as we have seen, this entire line of reasoning is false.

Weight stigma affects everyone, not just larger people. Naturally slender people who are terrified of gaining weight develop anxiety and disordered relationships with food and their own bodies. Poor body image and food anxiety impact relationships, so other people are affected as well. It is nearly impossible to be comfortable in an intimate relationship when you constantly feel shame about your body.

Another complicated concept is *thin privilege*. As with any other kind of privilege, the people who have it are generally unaware of it until it is pointed out to them. It is quite possible to benefit from thin privilege and still have poor body image, anxiety regarding food, and disordered eating. However, it is still important to acknowledge that weight stigma affects people differently, depending on their actual body size.

Here are some questions to help think about thin privilege:

- Have you ever dreaded going to a public place because you did not know whether you could fit in the seats?
- Have you ever wondered whether your doctor's office has a blood pressure cuff big enough for your arm?
- Have you ever worried about other people's reactions when you get on a plane or other public transport?
- Have you ever avoided exercising in public because of experiences of being mooed at from a car?
- Have you ever had a stranger criticize what is in your cart at the grocery store?
- Have you ever avoided a family gathering because of relatives who lecture you about weight loss "for your own good"?
- Have you ever had a medical professional ignore your concerns and talk about diets instead?
- Have you ever had a server in a restaurant bring you a diet soda when you ordered a regular soda because he assumed that is what you intended?

I could go on and on, but you get the picture. Weight stigma damages everyone, but it is much more direct and overt for fat people. It is also intersectional, in that it plays out differently depending on other identities, such as race, gender, disability, ethnicity, socioeconomic status, and age. *Intersectionality* refers to the ways that individuals are identified and characterized and how those categories combine to produce power differentials, inclusion or exclusion, privilege or marginalization. Body size is highly visible and is often an important criteria when bodies are being judged.[1] Addressing the intersectionality of weight stigma is beyond the scope of this book, but I do want to acknowledge it.

Weight stigma can be internal or external, obvious or stealthy. It can be deliberate or unconscious. External weight oppression, such as bullying, is often internalized. The person being bullied agrees with the bully: "There is something wrong with me. I deserve this." In fact, shaming someone about weight is often seen as something positive because of the mistaken idea that it will motivate change.

Many kinds of stigma and prejudice exist in the world. With other forms of oppression and discrimination, there is usually a sense of righteous anger at being treated badly for a characteristic or identity. There may also be a sense of belonging, even pride, about membership in the group, such as the black pride movement or gay rights parades. Internalized weight stigma is more damaging when there is no sense of community identity to buffer the effects.

Another way of thinking about this is the concept of in-group and reference group.[2] The *in-group* is where one belongs or feels a sense of membership. The *reference group* is the one that is accepted, acceptable, and has obvious advantages. The reference group might be rich people, white people, able-bodied people, straight people, male people, or people who belong to a certain club or attend a certain school; everyone else is excluded. Sometimes group membership can be changed: poor people can imagine becoming rich, and nonmembers can join a club. Other times, membership cannot be changed or individuals would not choose to change if they could: people of color cannot become white, and gay people may or may not wish they could become straight. In any case, there is recognition that being a member of the reference group has certain benefits, but membership in the in-group may offer benefits as well. Members of in-groups can, together, refuse to accept a devalued status, can reclaim derogatory terms, can offer community support, and can, collectively, challenge discrimination. Membership in the in-group can help buffer the effects of stigma and discrimination.

Weight stigma may be unique in the way it fits this model. Statistically, two-thirds of the population belongs to the in-group defined as "overweight/obese." Most of the remainder feels that they are at risk of being in the in-group or believe that they are, in fact, already there. In this case, the reference group is defined as thin and healthy, usually young, white, and conventionally attractive. Practically no one considers themselves as a member of the reference group. Of the tiny percentage of people who appear to others to fit the narrow definition, most have their own body image and eating insecurities that prevent them from enjoying the privilege that the world bestows on them.

Meanwhile, advantages of membership in an in-group are lost when everyone is trying to move out of it. When people find their way to a body positive group, or a Health At Every Size forum, or a Fat Acceptance gathering, the support they find has a stigma-buffering effect that can be hugely beneficial if they are able to acknowledge and accept their membership.

The words we use matter. They shape the way we think. The words that are used to talk about weight carry negative judgments and are stigmatizing in and of themselves. *Obese* implies disease and diagnosis, something that is outside the norm. *Overweight* implies that there is a proper weight that should not be exceeded. The term *morbidly obese* carries an enormous amount of negative judgment. Euphemisms such as *fluffy* or *queen-sized* also carry a negative connotation because we use euphemisms for things that are unpleasant, undesirable, or impolite to discuss. Certainly the F-word, *fat*, makes people uncomfortable.

The practice of person-first language originated with disability advocates as a way to address stigma. Many organizations now encourage the phrasing "person with a disability" as preferable to "disabled person." Weight-focused research journals encourage this, preferring "a person with obesity" or "person living with obesity" rather than "obese person." Other advocates, however, point out the ways that person-first language reinforces stigma, because, in practice, it is used to describe characteristics that are considered negative or undesirable. For instance, it may seem nicer to refer to a student as "a child with autism" until you realize that you never hear about "a child with neuro-typicalness." Furthermore, a tall person is not likely to be referred to as "a person with tallness."[3] When it comes to weight, there is a wide range of descriptors, all of which have different meanings to different people. What words do you want to use or choose to use that will contribute to your sense of self-worth?

Ragen Chastain, the author of *Fat: The Owner's Manual*[4] and the blog *DancesWithFat*, tells of arranging to meet someone for the first time and describing herself: "I'll be the short fat brunette." The other person often says, "Oh, you shouldn't call yourself fat!" They never say, "You shouldn't call yourself short" or "You shouldn't call yourself brunette." Words matter.

For Shame!

We take better care of what we love than what we hate.

—Peggy Elam[5]

One area of attention in the field of public health focuses on large-scale efforts to get people to make good health decisions, whether they want to or not. Sometimes this has to do with legislation, like traffic tickets for not wearing a seat belt, and sometimes it targets individual choices. In some situations, the deliberate use of shame has been found to be an effective agent of change. For instance, when I was a child, no one paid much attention if someone drove a car after drinking alcohol; now that behavior is framed as shameful and is much less common. Similarly, cigarette smoking has decreased, in part, because of campaigns to shame people who smoke in public. Because of this, many people, including the general public as well as medical and public health professionals, think that shame is an acceptable and effective, even desirable, intervention to deal with the alleged "obesity epidemic."

There are several problems with this approach, not the least of which is that it does not work, and it is just mean. Cigarette smoking, seat belt wearing, and drunk driving are all behaviors that can be changed. Weight is a characteristic that, as we have seen, is extremely difficult and unlikely to be altered. As we reviewed in chapter 2, shame and stigma do not lead to weight loss. In fact, there is considerable evidence that weight-shaming correlates to increased disordered eating and depression and decreased engagement in healthy behaviors such as exercise or fruit and vegetable intake.[6-9]

According to Brene Brown, "Shame is the intensely painful feeling or experience of believing we are flawed and therefore unworthy of acceptance and belonging."[10] Stigma is about cultural and societal values, while shame is personal. Shame that is a result of internalized weight stigma is debilitating and unnecessary. Human beings are worthy of acceptance and belonging simply because we exist. We do not have to meet an unreasonable societal standard to prove our worth.

While men can certainly suffer from body shame, almost all women have dealt with it at some level. Some years ago, I attended a lecture about women and art. The take-home moment for me was when the speaker said, "When you see a woman depicted in art, is she the object of the male gaze, or is she the subject of her own life?" This is a powerful question. We all want to be the subject of our own lives, but our culture teaches us that a woman's worth is based on her ability to draw the male gaze. This is so pervasive that it is rarely questioned. The "ideal" is impossible to attain, yet the quest for it is nearly impossible to relinquish. The inevitable failure to achieve the ideal reinforces shame.

How do we change this in ourselves? The first step is recognizing it, and the second is making a choice to be different. With time and determination, we can stop, or at least reduce, the impact that it has in our lives.

However much time and energy we focus on what we look like is less time and energy we have for other things. Turning toward our lives requires turning away from the mirror. When we use up our cognitive resources monitoring our bodies, we have less belief in our ability to be effective in the world.

When we consider ourselves as objects to be viewed, we undermine our own ability to identify our internal states of hunger, fullness, fatigue, or distress. For more on this concept, see Renee Engeln's book *Beauty Sick*.[11]

Informed Choices

When making a decision to approach eating and health differently, it is common to encounter those who want to argue with our choices. I had an interesting experience a couple of years ago when I responded to an article in the local paper that had been written by a personal trainer in another state. The paper included her name and email address, so I opened a cyberconversation, particularly about her assertion that "eating less than the body needs will result in weight loss, plain and simple." I sent links to some of the research articles that support the idea that the body has ways to maintain the set point in the face of dietary restriction, and she sent me links to articles about the Weight Control Registry (a resource that has had its validity questioned by many researchers). We had a lively exchange, but it became clear that neither one of us was going to change the other's mind. She truly believed that anyone could become thin with enough determination and perseverance, and she was unwilling to consider any evidence to the contrary. Ultimately, she believed that it was wrong for me to "steal people's dreams" of eventually being thin; I believed that it was wrong for her to encourage a dream that was impossible for the vast majority of the people who pursued it and would likely harm most of them in the process.

In contrast, about that same time, a young woman in my area was preparing to compete, for the second time, in the Olympic Trials in pole vault. I live in a small town. Thus, the local news followed her endeavors closely, and she received much support from the community. It occurred to me that there might be some parallels between what this trainer was recommending for weight loss and qualifying for the Olympics. The young pole-vaulter certainly had plenty of determination and perseverance as well as a small chance for success. The difference was that she knew going into the process that her chance for success was limited. She had a very clear idea of how hard she would have to train, what other activities she would have to give up, what sacrifices she would have to make, and how long it would take. She knew there was a risk of injury every time she left the ground and returned to it. She knew her chances of making the team were very small and not entirely under her control. No matter how hard she worked or how determined she was, there could still be three other women who would jump higher.

The big difference is that she made an informed decision. She knew the risks and chances when she made the commitment to try. Weight loss approaches that focus on determination and perseverance without providing information about the physical and emotional risks and miniscule likelihood of success are an enormous disservice to the very people they claim to be encouraging.

The woman who wrote the article thought I was wrong for stealing people's dreams of being thin. When people put their entire lives on hold while they pursue an impossible goal while constantly berating themselves for being inadequate, they are having their lives stolen, and I think that is much worse.

Making Changes

She understood that the hardest times in life to go through were when you were transitioning from one version of yourself to another.
—Sarah Addison Allen, from *Lost Lake*[12]

When you make the choice to give up the impossible goal of weight loss and choose instead to focus on your own well-being, expect to get a lot of push back from people in your life. Among other things, you will be accused of "giving up" on yourself. What exactly are you giving up? You are giving up repeated failure, you are giving up living in a perpetual sense of shame, and you are giving up harming yourself. You are embracing self-esteem, good self-care, and an improved quality of life. You are embracing a healthier life-style. You are embracing you!

This does not mean it will be easy. People around you will argue and harangue you about weight loss. You get to decide, situation by situation, how to respond. Some days, you may have enough energy to present the new information you have learned and perhaps you can influence someone. Other days, you may choose to smile, nod, and change the subject. It is always your choice how to react and how to take care of yourself (see Underpants Rule). Just remember, it is the focus on weight loss that causes suffering, not the weight itself.

Linda originally came to me for therapy for her anxiety, which was interfering with her ability to go to work each day. We focused on anxiety management techniques for several sessions before she mentioned her crippling sense of failure about her weight. As a chubby child, she started her first diet in grade school, with her unsuccessful attempts at weight loss becoming a defining dynamic of her life. She was a classic example of someone who was eating nutritiously and exercising regularly but was still heavy. Over time, we explored the ideas and information about normalizing eating and questioning the assumptions about weight that had influenced her. Her anxiety did not disappear, but it was considerably diminished when she relinquished her goal of weight loss.

Linda's husband, however, continued to nag at her, and he refused to even consider any of the articles she suggested that he read. At one point in this process, she told me that she had signed up for a commercial online weight loss program; as long as her husband saw the automatic payment from the bank account each month, he assumed she was following the program and left her alone about it. While I do not advocate lying to one's husband, it was her choice, and this gave her enough time to become more confident about her decision. She stopped trying to change him, and, with practice, she eventually became quite adept at ignoring him when he made comments about her weight. Eventually, she was able to have more assertive conversations with him about how her resentment of his attitude was affecting their relationship, and he (mostly) stopped nagging. She was able to make decisions about her own life and behavior, even as her husband violated the Underpants Rule.

Choosing how to respond to people who make weight-stigmatizing comments is another opportunity to think about the message you give yourself about your own worth. Having some phrases ready helps prevent freezing in the moment and regretting it later. Obviously, appropriate responses change with the context. You would not say the same thing to your elderly grandmother as you might say to a judgmental stranger in the grocery store, but thinking ahead helps.

An all-purpose response that is handy in many situations, weight related and otherwise, is, "Why would you think it's okay to say that?" This puts the responsibility back on the speaker and gives you a moment to think. It is equally effective when the problematic comment is directed at you, when it is about someone else, or when the speaker is talking about themselves. Depending on the tone of voice, it can be genuinely curious or confrontational.

I recently had an interesting conversation with a young man who works as a barista in a coffee shop in a university town. He asked me to suggest appropriate responses when a customer makes a self-disparaging comment when ordering. He was quite distressed at some of the hateful things he heard women say about themselves. He understood that replying with a variation of, "But you are beautiful," was unacceptable on several levels, including the fact that it reinforced the standard that beauty is more important than anything else. We discussed more general comments, such as "I wish we lived in a world where everyone could feel happy with their bodies" or "Wouldn't it be nice if we could all appreciate our bodies more for what they do than how they look?" or even "I think we all deserve to enjoy food without guilt." Eventually, he came up with his own favorite response to customers randomly telling him about their diets or weight concerns: "Oh no, dude, dieting and weightism is the patriarchy—down with patriarchy!"

In social situations, weight loss is often a topic of discussion. Comments like "I prefer to talk about other things than body size" might work or simply changing the subject, "How about them Cards?" (Although, "How about them Cards?" might only work in St. Louis.) If it feels more personal, a statement such as "I'm working on a weight-neutral approach based on the Health At Every Size principles; would you like to hear about it?" might help. If someone is really trying to push their weight loss propaganda on you, consider saying, "I know you are trying to help. What you are doing is not helpful to me. It would be more helpful to me if we could go on a walk together and talk about something else." Or say, "Please stop. If you cannot stop, I will end this conversation," and be prepared to do so. If a conversation is triggering or toxic for you, the best thing you can do for yourself is get out of it.

When you become more comfortable with living your life without pursuing weight loss, you may find that speaking out feels empowering. Recently, Christina, a young woman who is well into her recovery for an eating disorder but still sees me occasionally to talk about family issues, shared an example with me. She had been approached on social media by a couple of different women who were selling their services as Beachbody coaches with advice about diet and exercise. Christina proudly told me that, instead of simply ignoring them, she fired back a message about how they were promoting disordered eating behavior and weight stigma. She did not know whether she changed their minds, but she felt powerful in speaking her truth and strong in her own recovery.

People who speak out publicly, especially on social media, about accepting body diversity and the other principles supported by the Health At Every Size approach are often accused of "glorifying obesity." Whenever members of a marginalized group push for equal treatment, there is a likelihood that members of the dominant group will see that as a threat. The response is usually unrealistic and poorly considered. This dynamic has been evident throughout the women's movement, as many men feel that they are being unfairly targeted, and in the movement for racial justice, when those who benefit from inequality are the most likely to become defensive. Sometimes the pushback focuses on exaggerated threats, such as when people who ask for the benefits of same-sex marriage are accused of trying to turn children into homosexuals. The idea of "glorifying obesity" falls into this category.

Promoting body diversity is hardly glorifying any particular size. Conversely, "glorifying thinness" promotes stigma and discrimination. My own thoughts are that the people most likely to worry about glorifying obesity are those who have invested a huge amount of time and energy in trying to suppress their own weight; they are terrified that if they stop, they will binge and gain weight forever. That is their own problem, not mine or yours. If someone says this to you, consider your options. You can walk away or you can ask them to explain. You can keep asking questions, or not, because Underpants Rule. You may or may not change their thinking, but you can set limits on how you will interact.

Ahimsa

One of the *yamas*, or ethical principles of yoga, is ahimsa, which means nonviolence. This is not just about physical violence toward others; it also includes our words and thoughts about others and about ourselves. It is about acting with compassion and clarity toward ourselves and others in everyday activities and in response to anything that is dangerous or threatening. My yoga teacher sometimes uses the phrase "Don't get combative with it" when teaching a particularly challenging pose. Sometimes she will stop students from trying when she sees that they are getting angry with themselves for not achieving the full expression of the posture. She teaches that honoring ahimsa is more important than attaining some arbitrary goal.

How often does your internal dialog violate the principles of ahimsa? How often do you have conversations with others that reinforce a sense of shame and inadequacy? Harriet Brown[13] refers to the "call and response" of the common pattern of negative body talk, which goes something like this: "I can't believe I ate that; I'm so bad!" then "What do you mean you're so bad? I'm worse!" with infinite variations. This kind of conversation is so widespread that is goes without notice, but it is very harmful. On the surface, it sounds supportive and reassuring, but it actively reinforces objectification and shame. Studies have shown that many women feel expected to participate in these conversations to be considered acceptable.[14] It is expected, as if it is some kind of bonding ritual. Renee Engeln's research clearly shows that negative body talk is not comforting or supportive; instead, it increases body dissatisfaction and shame.[15,16] Even overhearing it increases body monitoring. It violates ahimsa. It is verbal and emotional violence against oneself and against the others involved. What can we do instead?

Again, the first step is to notice and identify it when it happens. There are a number of ways to respond, and you get to choose what to do in any given situation (see Underpants Rule). When your best friend says, "Ugh, my thighs are so huge," you could respond with, "It makes me sad to hear you talk about yourself like that"; "Is something bothering you that you'd like to talk about?"; "I'm trying to develop a worldview that places less emphasis on appearance"; or "I heard it might snow tomorrow." My personal favorite is, "Hey, I'm reading this really great book about how appearance is objectified in culture and what we can do about it!"

It may be more challenging to deal with this when it is happening in your own head, but changes in the way you talk to yourself are powerful. Objectification is about appearance. What happens when you shift focus to function instead? Can you think of all the wonderful things your body does? Can you imagine thanking your body for them? Right now, this minute, your brain is processing these words. Your heart is pumping blood to that very same brain, taking it the oxygen and energy it needs to do its job. Your lungs, without any conscious command from you, are absorbing that very oxygen. Once you start thinking this way, you will never run out of things to be thankful to your body for.

Years ago, when I worked in the eating disorder treatment program, one of the group activities involved a handout with open-ended questions and instructions to answer them with examples of function rather than appearance. It was a fun group and often yielded surprising results. You can try it.

Body Questionnaire

I love my arms because _____.
I love my hips because _____.
I love my eyes because _____.
I love my feet because _____.
I love my hands because _____.
I love my knees because _____.
I love my brain because _____.
I love my lips because _____.
I love my belly because _____.
I love my ears because _____.

The answers are often delightful, such as "I love my arms because I can hug my mom with them," or "I love my hips because I can carry my baby sister on them," or "I love my lips because they allow me to form words to name the oppression I see in the world."

Another helpful activity is to keep a variation on a gratitude journal. Each day, write down three things that you appreciate about your body's ability to function. Perhaps engage a friend and do it together or make a commitment to each other to do it daily. Eventually, these statements become useful in dealing with negative body talk. When someone says, "Ugh, I hate my fat thighs," you are prepared with a response: "I love my thighs because they are strong and help me lift heavy things without putting a strain on my back."

Consider your closet. Dieting mentality teaches us to save our too-small clothes in the hopes that we can get back into them. This is shaming and a violation of ahimsa, nonviolence. You deserve to have clothing that fits and makes you feel good. Think about the items in your wardrobe that make you feel bad about yourself and let go of them. Send them back out into the river of life; donate them or take them to a consignment store.

The ways we compliment other people also reflect and reinforce our values regarding bodies. "You look great! Have you lost weight?" is a very common comment, intended to be a compliment, that highlights the assumptions and myths we have been talking about. Sometimes referred to as *thin praising*, it seems nice on the surface but is the flip side of fat shaming. By definition, any message that glorifies thinness stigmatizes fatness. Any compliment about appearance is also a reminder that appearance is being monitored and evaluated. How many other ways can we think of to compliment others by focusing on something other than appearance? Examples might include, "You did a great job on that presentation; I'm glad we are on the same team," or "I appreciate that you are so quick to lend a hand," or "Your comments in that discussion gave me some new insight, thanks!" The more you offer creative positive feedback to others, the more you will internalize the concept for yourself.

Many people are conflicted about taking in compliments, even when it is intended to be relatively neutral feedback. Lisa is rather delightful young woman who initially came to me for treatment of depression. Her family of origin still operates on the principle that any kind of praise leads to conceit and arrogance. Because of this, she has very clear ideas of all the things that are wrong with her, a limited ability to see her own assets, and a very low sense of self-worth. On several occasions, she has become tearful in response to a comment from me that she considers a "compliment" that I intended as neutral feedback. She is slowly practicing accepting comments that are other than negative and critical.

The proper response to a compliment is, "Thank you." We all know that, but the fear of appearing conceited creates a double bind. If you routinely dismiss and contradict positive feedback, it may be worthwhile to pay attention and see whether you can practice a different response. It is an opportunity to learn and grow.

Let's Detox!

The world is full of suggestions about ways to "detox" or "cleanse" your body. These suggestions have limited to no scientific evidence, and they reinforce body dissatisfaction while claiming to promote good self-care. But what about a media cleanse? Or a bad body talk detox?

Once you have developed the ability to identify your own bad body thoughts, they can guide you in making decisions. We talked about this when evaluating options for physical activity. What media do you consume? Often, the images that we allow into our heads are just as influential as the food we put into our mouths. It we do not eat toxic food, why would we consume toxic images and media? How can we avoid it?

Consider an audit of the media and images that you consume. What messages do they give you about your own worth? We have known for decades that time spent reading fashion magazines correlates with increased body dissatisfaction. Today, thanks to social media, we have infinitely more opportunities to be exposed to unrealistic images and information that make us feel bad. You can learn to manage this.

We learned in chapter 4 that we can improve our ability to respond to an internal locus of control until it is a habit when we are eating. We do this by paying attention to internal signals and cues, especially regarding hunger and satiety. This same principle applies to images and information. An increase in bad body thoughts is valuable data. It means that something important is happening, and you can learn from it. If you are watching a movie or following a Twitter thread and notice thoughts like "I should really go on a diet; I'm disgusting," stop and ask, "What just happened?" Remember that the purpose of most media is to sell us a product by making us feel bad about ourselves. We do not have to participate.

Stop watching shows that increase bad body thoughts. Curate your social media. Delete pages, blogs, or accounts that promote dieting and weight stigma. Trust your own intuition, your own internal locus of control.

As Anthony Warner says, "The end goal of all eating should not be a good-looking Instagram shot. The pleasure of eating should be embraced for what it is: variety, joy, precious moments shared."[17]

We can stop blaming our bodies for the meanness of the world.

"Everyone Is Beautiful in Their Own Way"

When did being beautiful become more important than anything else? When did beauty become the quality that is desired above all others? When did "No, you're not fat; you're beautiful" become the default response for offering comfort?

The very word *beauty* is complicated. It means that something is pleasing to the senses (sunsets, flowers, the sound of a baby laughing), but it is increasingly used to refer to a narrowly defined, culturally determined physical appearance. It is disproportionately used in conversations about women. It is objectifying and reinforces stigma.

I have been doing a (very unscientific) study for some time now while scrolling through Facebook. If a female-identifying person posts a picture, any kind of picture, most of the responses will be some variation on "Beautiful!" When a male-identifying person posts a picture, the comments are rarely about how he looks, focusing instead on what he is doing or where he is. What would it be like to live in a world that focused on activities and abilities rather than appearance?

When the word *beautiful* is used, can you take a moment and reflect on it? Does it describe something other than a person's appearance, such as a song? Or is it being used to comfort someone by affirming that they have worth? Think about it. Pay attention. Words matter.

I was recently introduced to the concept of *beauty privilege*. The woman who was called out on it was surprised and taken aback, as she had never considered herself attractive. She had internalized the impossible cultural standards of beauty and had given up on ever achieving them. She was oblivious to her own loveliness. What defines conventional physical beauty? It involves symmetrical features that are in proportion to one another, although how those features are valued changes historically and culturally. Whether a face has pronounced cheekbones or is round, whether lips are slight or full, whether noses are narrow or wide are preferences that are imbedded in cultural constructs. The skin on women's faces is expected to be smooth, while men can be craggier. Large eyes are considered attractive in women, but less important in men.

Having some level of conventional beauty in a culture carries with it certain privileges and limits. A conventionally attractive person may be more likely to be listened to (especially when talking to a reporter who has brought along a photographer) but less likely to be taken seriously when expressing controversial views. Even acknowledging the existence of beauty privilege is conflicted. To recognize one's own pleasant appearance is considered conceited and arrogant. Accepting one's attractiveness makes one unattractive. There is no way to get it right!

This is also noticeable when women talk about being photographed, a phenomenon that has increased now that nearly everyone has a cell phone with the capacity to effortlessly take and share photos. The tendency to find fault with our own image seems amplified along with the number of images. Pamela is a middle-aged women who has made great strides in dealing with an eating disorder, but she still struggles with depression. Because she is on disability, it is easy for her to withdraw from social interaction and become isolated; she knows she needs to push herself to participate in friendly gatherings. We discussed why this was particularly challenging over the winter holidays this past year. "I knew everyone would be taking pictures, and I'm so ugly!" As is true for many women, she overestimates the importance of her features and underestimates her likeability. We talked about the warmth and delight that we feel when we see a picture of someone we care about on social media, without regard to their actual appearance. I encouraged her to think about the joy that her friends could experience when seeing her picture.

How do we change the conversation? Sarah is a young woman who fulfills the current cultural definition of beauty. She has made great strides in her work with me in overcoming her eating disorder, but she still struggles with body image. "I know better!" she lamented to me recently, acknowledging the power of the societal pressures to attain an impossible ideal and the difficulty in resisting. She struggled to change a lifelong habit of comparing herself to other women. "When I walk into a room, I still look around to see how many women are prettier than me." We discussed what to do instead and other adjectives and descriptors to use. In a room full of strangers, she could look around to see who looks interesting, appealing, intriguing, lonely, wise, uncomfortable, confident, shy, friendly, kind, or unconventional. She could then challenge herself to approach someone and start a conversation and see whether her initial perception was accurate. In our discussion, we compared the process of discovering how to enjoy food again instead of missing out with the possibility of finding new friends she might have missed out on by only focusing on "beauty."

Defining What Is Wrong

Dr. Beverly Crusher was a character on the science fiction television program *Star Trek: The Next Generation*. One episode, "Remember Me," which aired in 1990, featured a plot in which she gets trapped, unknowingly, in a "warp bubble," and everyone and everything around her is disappearing. She explores all the possible reasons, including her own sanity, and rejects them all. Beverly then says, "If there's nothing wrong with me, maybe there's something wrong with the universe." If you find yourself thinking that, perhaps, you should reconsider and go back to trying to change your weight to make other people happy, remind yourself this: There is nothing wrong with you! There is something wrong with the universe!

Whatever decisions you make for your own life, we still live in a world that believes certain falsehoods: that weight is mutable, that shame is motivating, and that health is an obligation. It is not your responsibility to educate others about it, although you may if you choose. Some days you may have enough energy to challenge the falsehoods; other days, you will not. That is okay. You get to decide to live in the way that works best for you, because Underpants Rule.

In the next chapter, we are going to look at stigma and the research about it on a broader scale, as it applies to policy, discrimination, and society.

CHAPTER SEVEN

Social Justice: Weight Stigma, Part 2

What do we mean when we talk about *social justice*? It is a multifaceted concept that recognizes that not all people have access to the same social benefits, opportunities, rights, and protections; that all people deserve them; and that there are ways to address these disparities. *Equality* means treating everyone the same, while *equity* recognizes that not everyone starts in the same place; not everyone needs the same help. The goal of social justice is for everyone to have what they need to participate in society, reach their full potential, and thrive. Social justice requires recognizing and addressing discrimination and oppression, including when it is caused by weight stigma.

People who work in the field of public health often talk about *upstream* or *downstream* interventions and outcomes, referring to treating a problem versus preventing it. There are different versions of a story to explain this, and I would like to share mine.

A group of friends were having a picnic one sunny afternoon on the banks of a river. Suddenly, someone said, "Look! There is someone in the water!" Sure enough, there was a person struggling against the current. The friends organized themselves and pulled the wet and shivering individual out of the flow, wrapped her in a blanket and asked, "What happened?" The reply was, "Someone pushed me into the water!" They looked out at the river and cried, "There is someone else! And another! And another!" Soon they all focused on pulling people out of the current. No one had time to go upstream to see who was pushing them into the river and make them stop.

Weight stigma has pushed us all into the river. Promoting body insecurity allows the highly profitable weight loss industry to continue making money.

Weight stigma distracts from other social concerns, such as racism, classism, sexism, and all other systems that promote a hierarchy of one kind of people as better than another. Weight stigma distracts from and interferes with efforts to promote a more fair and equitable society in which all people have access to health, security, and a better quality of life. Weight stigma is a medical issue, a public health issue, and a social justice issue.

Confirmation bias is the common tendency to embrace information that is familiar and that we agree with while rejecting information that challenges our beliefs. Our desires influence our beliefs; in other words, what do we want to be true? Reading this book has likely challenged your beliefs about eating, weight, health, and worthiness. Most of the rest of the world remains unconvinced.

Those who are comfortable with the status quo are less likely to challenge it. Those who are uncomfortable may find the tasks of challenging and changing it to be daunting and overwhelming, perhaps impossible. However, history shows us that social change can happen slowly and in small increments.

When talking about social change movements, I have a personal example. I graduated from college in the mid-1970s, and people smoked cigarettes everywhere. It was not unusual for a smoker to light up in someone else's car without asking. I remember the first time I met a person who was pushing back against that. I do not remember the organization he was with, but I remember that he gave me my first "Thank You for Not Smoking" sign. I asked him what I could do to help. He encouraged me to ask to be seated in the "nonsmoking section" every time I went to a restaurant, even if I already knew that they did not have one (many did not). For a couple of decades, I did just that. Then came the day, in the mid-1990s, when I was trying to corral my two young children into a restaurant in the Galleria Mall in St. Louis. I looked over my shoulder at the host and said, "Table for three, nonsmoking." He rolled his eyes and said something that sounded like "Pfft!" That was when I realized that the entire mall was nonsmoking! Small interventions over time lead to social change. Enough snowflakes become a blizzard.

There is a growing understanding among clinicians, researchers, activists, policy makers, and others that weight stigma is a social justice problem, a public health problem, and a quality of life problem. The more we raise awareness, the more we can plan change. We have to keep pulling people out of the river, but we also have to go upstream and stop weight stigma from pushing people into the water.

A. Janet Tomiyama et al. says, "We define weight stigma as the social rejection and devaluation that accrues to those who do not comply with prevailing social norms of adequate body weight and shape."[1] Weight stigma can be internal or external, implicit or explicit. It includes anything that shames or oppresses because of body size, anything that devalues larger bodies. It includes fatphobia, body dissatisfaction, stereotypes, unexamined assumptions, and institutionalized policy. It is used to justify and even encourage discrimination and oppression.

The word *stigma* comes from the Greek word that referred to a visible mark, such as a tattoo or scar, that identified someone as blemished or undesirable, someone to avoid. A stereotype assumes certain undesirable characteristics based on membership in a group. Social stigma is similar to stereotype, but it is generally associated with a visibly identifiable characteristic. For example, someone may hold stereotypical attitudes about members of a certain religion but not be able to identify those members based on a visual cue. Racial stereotypes, on the other hand, are more related to stigma because members of the group can usually be identified by visual characteristics. Weight stigma is not only based on visual cues but may differ in intensity based on how much a given person varies from the culturally dictated "ideal."

I have a few more words about words. Bias is a preconceived idea about something or someone that can be positive or negative, but the term is usually used to refer to a negative opinion. Stereotype is a belief, often supported by the culture, about people based on their membership in a group. Stereotypical ideas can serve as justification for behavior. Prejudice is a negative personal attitude, an unreasonable dislike of someone different from you. Bias, stereotypes, and prejudice are all attitudes that can be conscious or unconscious. It is possible to hold them without acting on them or even being aware of them.

Discrimination and oppression are behaviors that are based on prejudice and stereotype. Discrimination is negative, harmful, unjustified treatment based on preconceived judgment about a person's membership in a group. Oppression is systemic, the socially supported mistreatment and exploitation of a group of individuals, and it is dependent on power dynamics. Oppression requires a hierarchy, with a dominant group that benefits from authority and power, shaping life possibilities beyond personal control. Stigma and prejudice depend on social norms, while discrimination and oppression require actualization of negative judgment or behaviors toward the stigmatized target.

While weight stigma affects everyone, it has disproportionately negative impacts on those with less power in the social hierarchy, especially those who have other marginalized identities based on characteristics such as race, gender, sexual orientation, or physical ability, among others.

Types of Stigma

Interpersonal, or external, stigma is directed at other people. Intrapersonal, or internal, stigma is directed against oneself. Stigma can also be structural. Explicit stigma is expressed directly and clearly, leaving little room for doubt. Implicit stigma is implied and indirect, sometimes even unintentional.

Intrapersonal stigma occurs when an individual accepts as true a devalued identity based on membership in a group. In the case of weight stigma, an individual may accept the societal beliefs that her higher weight is a result of her own failures and shortcomings. She then believes that she deserves to be treated less well than a thinner person. When negative stereotypes about large people are endorsed and applied to oneself, it contributes to devaluing oneself.[2] She may or may not hold her own negative stereotypes about other fat people. These beliefs may be reinforced by anticipated stigma, when bad treatment is expected from other people. Internalized weight stigma results in feelings of guilt, shame, and worthlessness.

Body dissatisfaction and internalized weight stigma are related but different. Internalized weight stigma is often accompanied by obsessive negative thoughts about one's body and a relentless internal dialog of shaming and self-denigrating judgment. Body dissatisfaction can also exist when self-criticism and disparagement targets characteristics other than weight or size, such as (more often the case with men) a focus on being too small, too short, or lacking muscle. Self-blame is a large part of internalized weight stigma, while dissatisfaction can focus on specific body parts or features that are generally not perceived to be controllable.[3] For instance, a person may be very dissatisfied with his height but not feel guilty for causing it. Internalized weight stigma usually includes body dissatisfaction, but it is not the only reason for it.

Interpersonal, or external, stigma involves negative attitudes toward others based on their characteristics or membership in a group, in this case, the group of fat people. This can include overt discrimination, such as refusing to hire or promote fat people, or harassment, such as yelling obscenities at fat people from passing cars. Examples range from strangers commenting on food choices in restaurants or grocery stores to physical attacks. The practice of *concern trolling* involves judgmental comments that are framed as "for your own good." These comments come from friends, family members, coworkers, or strangers, but they all reinforce the idea that weight is a problem that needs to be fixed and can be fixed with the right information. Concern trolling seems, on the surface, to be caring, but it is, in fact, another type of socially acceptable bullying.

Structural stigma includes sociocultural norms and conditions and institutional policies that constrain the well-being of those stigmatized while reinforcing negative stereotypes. Examples of structural stigma include small seats in theaters and public transportation, equipment in medical facilities that does not fit larger bodies, and limited clothing sizes in brick-and-mortar stores. Policies that limit access to employment, rental property, medical care, insurance, immigration, or adoption all involve patterns of structural stigma. Structural stigma is rarely questioned; it is simply accepted as the norm, reinforcing bias and social acceptability.[4]

Social identity threat involves anticipated stigma and the risk of being badly treated for characteristics that are considered undesirable whether internalized stigma is present or absent.[5] In other words, whether or not an individual feels good about her body and rejects the stereotypes associated with her weight, she will still be aware of prevailing cultural attitudes. As an example, plus-sized model Tess Holliday was featured on the cover of *Cosmopolitan* magazine in October 2018. Although she is clearly comfortable in her own body and beauty, many online comments were angry, nasty, and abusive. However good she feels about her body, even when she rejects the cultural rhetoric about fatness, she will always be aware of the risks she takes by being unapologetically fat in the world.

Anticipated rejection because of body size is linked to impaired cognitive performance, anxiety, lower self-esteem, and rumination. It can lead to avoidance of situations because of anticipated stigma and rejection, which then affects employment, access to medical care, social relationships, and participation in society in general.[6]

Social identity threat exists even in the absence of enacted stigma; a person can experience it when alone because it is about expectation as well as experience. It leads to exhausting hypervigilance and chronic stress, which uses up cognitive resources and negatively affects health.[7] Even in the absence of self-devaluation, anticipated stigma can worsen internalization and have severe consequences.

The Acceptability of Stigma

Sociocultural norms influence how we feel about the acceptability and legitimacy of bias, stigma, and discrimination. Many people have a strong, negative, reflexive reaction to the suggestion of *discrimination*, as if it is always wrong and unacceptable. However, there are many types of discrimination that we do not question and many more that are the subject of debate.[8] We do not let 16-year-olds buy liquor, and we do not let noncitizens vote. Some discrimination has a legitimate basis in function; people with color blindness cannot be airplane pilots because they cannot tell the green lights from the blue ones.

The acceptability of discrimination changes over time. Things that we now find shocking were once commonplace, such as "Whites Only" drinking fountains or "No Indians Allowed" signs in parks. Most people born after 1958 or so do not even remember that the voting age used to be 21, which certainly discriminated against those old enough to be drafted at 18. Other types of discrimination continue to be matters of contention.

The concept of *mutability* refers to the ability to change. When characteristics are immutable, prejudice and discrimination are usually considered illegitimate, or at least socially unacceptable. Race, for instance, is immutable, and, in current polite society, most people deny feeling racial prejudice (even when they do). Even if they feel it, most people know that it is not socially acceptable behavior to openly express it in most situations. When a characteristic is considered a choice, attitudes about the legitimacy of discrimination are more variable and still historically changeable. For example, visible tattoos are more acceptable in the workplace than they were 30 years ago, and tattoos are clearly a choice. At the same time, blatant racial discrimination has been considered acceptable for much of human history, even though race is not mutable. Over time, the acceptability of racism is very slowly changing because it has been challenged over and over again. Historically, discriminatory attitudes against immutable characteristics, such as gender, physical disability, and even left-handedness, have changed only because they have been challenged.

Debates about the mutability or choice about characteristics can be contentious. The highly politicized dispute about same-sex marriage is a disagreement about the mutability of sexual orientation. One side of the question holds that heterosexuality is a choice that everyone can and should make, leading to the conclusion that certain rights and privileges should be denied to those who choose wrongly. This line of thought also leads to conversion therapy. The other side holds the belief that sexual orientation is not something we have control over and therefore should not be a reason for withholding the rights and privileges afforded to heterosexual individuals and couples from those who do not fit heteronormative expectations.

Another way of thinking about mutability is the social mobility belief system.[9] Are group membership boundaries permeable? Can a person leave the group? Can a person in a marginalized or disadvantaged group move into a more desirable group? A person without an education can become a college graduate. A poor person can, theoretically at least, become a rich person. If group boundaries are considered permeable, there is little motivation to try to improve the conditions for group members; instead, individuals focus on improving themselves. However, if group membership is not changeable, a sense of belonging can be a coping mechanism. Identifying with the group can lead to collectively challenging the status quo and committing to a social change strategy, which then leads to benefiting from the psychological resources of the group.

Discrimination, bias, and stigma regarding weight are based in beliefs about the mutability of body size. If weight can be changed through determination and willpower, then discrimination, shaming, and stigma are justified and socially sanctioned as motivation. However, science, research, and lived experience all support the conclusion that weight is not controllable by any sustainable means. The group membership boundaries are not permeable, yet a huge swath of the population invests enormous time, energy, and resources into trying to move out of the group. The benefits of group support and social change are voided when no one wants to claim membership. Instead, discrimination is seen as legitimate, even by members of the group.

Bias that is based on the belief that the stigmatized characteristic is controllable is perceived as socially acceptable, which influences cultural norms and expectations. Discriminatory and unfair treatment is more likely to be considered legitimate when group membership is seen as a choice.[10] Dismissing obesity as a result of personal failure increases the perception that stigma is acceptable while rationalizing discrimination, becoming justification for treating people badly. Internalized stigma and the social identity threat increase, creating a feedback loop.

Attitudes and bias can be either implicit or explicit. Explicit refers to the attitudes that we are aware of consciously, while implicit bias is unconscious, sometimes thought of as a "blind spot." Explicit attitudes may be related to social acceptability. It is possible to talk about equality for different groups, and even believe in those values, while still holding implicit, unconscious beliefs that differ. Harvard University has a website with tests to help people measure their own implicit bias, and the data collected there has revealed changes over time.[11] Between 2007 and 2016, implicit biases about race and sexual orientation have moved toward neutral but become more negative regarding weight.[12] Body size continues to be perceived as mutable and therefore the responsibility of the individual to "fix."

One of the challenges in researching and evaluating bias and prejudice is that some people may not express their true feelings because they do not want to appear to have socially unacceptable attitudes. This is less of a problem when the topic is body weight. Many individuals are quite willing to express their negative bias toward fat people, and they may even feel that it is obligatory.

Microaggressions are the subtle, sometimes unintentional, comments or actions that reinforce a bias or stereotype. They can cause insult or injury even when they do not reflect a malicious intent. They may be insults or invalidations. Anything that normalizes the devaluing of fat bodies is a microaggression based in weight stigma. By this definition, "Hey, you look great! Have you lost weight?" is a microaggression. The perpetrator of the microaggression may be unaware of it and become defensive when the behavior is identified. The response may be dismissive and invalidating: "You're too sensitive. You have no sense of humor. Don't take it personally." Microaggressions may also be a covert way to express prejudice when overt ways are unacceptable.

It is hard to live life when you always have to be prepared for bad treatment. It is exhausting to constantly be braced for microaggressions from television, movies, magazines, and people you meet. Microaggressions result in anticipated stigma, chronic stress, and hypervigilance, which are linked to health problems in and of themselves. Being able to recognize them for what they are, even when it is not possible to challenge them, can build resilience. When possible, limit exposure to them by avoiding certain media and, perhaps, certain people.

Weight stigma negatively affects more than just individuals. Health policy that focuses on weight loss ignores and obscures the effect of the social determinants of health. A wealth of information is available that shows that social class, income, gender, race, geography, and the conditions in which people live and work have more influence on health than personal behaviors or weight. For instance, poor people experience more stress, have less control over their lives, are more likely to live in areas with high levels of pollution, and have less access to health care than people who are more financially secure. The relationship between health and weight fades or disappears when controlling for social determinants of health. Addressing these important issues requires a shift in thinking, in social policy, and in funding. It is much easier to blame individual heavy people and their failures to reduce than it is to look at the larger picture and take responsibility for changing society.[13] More information about the social determinants of health can be found on the websites for the Centers for Disease Control and Prevention (CDC) and the World Health Organization (WHO) and in *The Health Gap*[14] and other writings of Sir Michael Marmot, a professor of epidemiology and public health at University College in London.

Weight bias influences our society and culture in many ways, large and small. When it comes to designing research, policy, practice, public health interventions, and antidiscrimination legislation, large people are not involved, are marginalized, or are ignored. The (usually slender) people designated as experts choose directions and methods without considering the lived experiences of the people they are trying to change. Meanwhile, weight bias is increasing among those very experts.[15]

Let's revisit Allport, Clark, and Pettigrew's seminal book on prejudice, *The Nature of Prejudice*, mentioned in the previous chapter and their terminology of *in-group* and *reference group*.[16] The in-group is where one belongs, the we/us. The reference group is the one that is warmly accepted and has obvious advantages; it is the group that one aspires to and in which one wishes to be included. In the case of weight and body size, the reference group is the thin, "healthy," and beautiful people we see in magazines, movies, and television. The in-group is basically everyone else. No one wants to be in the in-group, but almost no one belongs to the reference group. Those who do belong to the reference group may not believe that they belong or are terrified of gaining weight or aging and moving out of the reference group. Meanwhile, there is no stigma-buffering effect of membership in the in-group if no one claims membership in it: "You can't advocate for yourself if you won't admit what you are."[17]

Group membership, identification, and support can buffer the negative impacts of stigma, but it requires the belief that the stigma is not legitimate.[18] Relinquishing attempts to move out of the in-group through weight loss allows access to the benefits of group membership. Increased identity with the marginalized group can counteract some of the harm caused by discrimination. Group membership influences positive social identities while providing social support for dealing with discrimination and stigma, leading to a range of positive impacts on physical and mental health.[19]

A sense of belonging is an important coping mechanism. Identifying with a group can lead to social change strategies and collectively challenging the status quo. Benefiting from the psychological resources of the group requires claiming group membership.[20] The sense of safety in group membership increases a sense of worth and belonging while decreasing the need for hypervigilance, all of which help cope with stigma.[21]

As Lindy West says, "That's why reclaiming fatness—living visibly, declaring 'I'm fat and I am not ashamed'—is a social tool so revolutionary, so liberating, it saves lives."[22]

Health Effects of Stigma

When weight stigma is internalized, it leads to shame and poor body image. It has also been shown to correlate with increased disordered eating, decreased healthy behaviors, and worse health measures, such as metabolic syndrome. The very problems that are blamed on weight may, instead, be caused by weight stigma. When the stress of living with the external weight stigma that we experience in the world, especially in medical settings, is added, the effects grow.

A large and growing body of literature supports the idea that weight stigma is, in and of itself, harmful to health. It is related to increased stress, with its associated negative effects on health; unhealthy behavior changes, including disordered eating; decreased access to medical care; and social disconnection.[23]

Stress takes a toll on the body. The experience of both acute and chronic stress in response to interpersonal weight stigma is related to poorer physical health measures, including hypertension, cardiovascular problems, diabetes, and overall impaired health.[24] Repeated experiences of weight discrimination are significantly correlated to increased cortisol (stress hormone) and oxidative stress, independent of actual body weight. High levels of cortisol are associated with increased blood pressure, insulin resistance, and an impaired immune response.[25] It is likely that many of the health problems commonly associated with obesity are, in fact, related to stress caused by stigma.[26] Eradicating weight stigma would improve health for everyone because it causes harm to everyone, across the BMI spectrum.[27]

Weight Stigma and Medical Care

Medical professionals are not immune to the cultural attitudes about weight. In fact, weight bias has been specifically marketed to doctors by the companies that profit from selling weight loss drugs and products.[28] When the quality of care that is provided is compromised by weight stigma, health is directly undermined.[29] This becomes a structural form of enacted stigma when it negatively affects the quality of care given to heavier people, making them reluctant to access needed medical care in the future.

Avoidance of medical care in heavier people is well documented.[30] Large women who delayed or avoided recommended cancer screenings reported that the barriers to accessing care included negative attitudes of providers, disrespectful treatment, unpleasant experiences with being weighed, equipment that is too small, and unsolicited advice about weight loss. Women of higher body weight reported these concerns more often. Women who had been on more weight loss programs were more likely to delay care.[31] When fat people do access health care, they are less likely to receive evidence-based, bias-free medical care.[32]

Experienced and internalized weight stigma are related to body-related shame and guilt, and health care stress associated with body-related shame contributes to health care avoidance. Heavier women are then less likely to seek health care than thinner women.[33]

Fat people are less likely to access health care, including preventative screenings, even after controlling for other factors that are usually implicated, such as socioeconomic status or lack of health insurance. When patients feel disrespected by their medical providers, not taken seriously, and blamed for their problems because of their weight, they avoid the doctor's office. Weight stigma leads to substandard care and compromises health.[34]

In the summer of 2018, the obituary for Ellen Maud Bennett was reposted widely on the Internet. She passed away at the age of 64 after being diagnosed with inoperable cancer only days before. She had been feeling unwell for several years, but when she sought out medical intervention, the only recommendation given to her was weight loss. Her family asked that her story be shared widely, as her dying wish was to encourage women of size to advocate for themselves and not accept that fat is the only important health issue. She wanted to share a message about fat shaming in the medical profession. Weight stigma killed her.[35]

Unfortunately, this is not an isolated incident. Members of online groups share endless stories about being misdiagnosed and undertreated when weight is blamed for anything and everything. Additionally, sometimes a diagnosis of cancer is delayed because the symptom of weight loss is greeted with approval and praise.

Many years ago, when I worked on an inpatient psychiatric unit, I stopped by a patient's room to see whether she wanted to meet with me. She sat sobbing on the bed. She told me that the internal medicine resident had just been to see her and had yelled at her for not following her diabetic diet after she asked why her ankles were so swollen. She sobbed, "I have been following it! I only use a couple of grains of sugar in my coffee, to cut the taste of the NutraSweet!" She pointed to her ankles, which were so swollen that the skin was beginning to crack. I went to the nurses' station to look at her chart. This was back in the day when all charting was done on paper; the patients were weighed three times a week, but the results were recorded on a separate page each time. No one had noticed that she had gained 17 pounds in one week. I walked over to the head nurse and silently pointed to the information. Without speaking, she went to the phone and called the admitting psychiatrist. Within an hour, the patient was in an operating room having several liters of water drained from her chest. She nearly died of congestive heart failure because of the resident's unexamined assumptions and weight stigma.

Cultural weight stigma is implicated in the development of eating disorders, which are the psychiatric diagnostic category with the highest mortality rate. However, even people who work in the eating disorder treatment field are not immune to weight bias.[36] This bias affects both treatment and diagnosis. Recovery from an eating disorder is based on improvement in symptoms, but it is often measured by weight restoration. The stereotypical patient with anorexia nervosa is noticeably and dramatically underweight, and treatment goals usually include reaching a "normal" weight as defined by BMI. Depending on the individual and her natural set point, this may not be enough. Some individuals who started at a higher weight need to restore to that weight to recover from the behavioral aspects of the illness, but treatment may emphasize an arbitrary "healthy weight," which reinforces weight suppression.[37]

The newest version of the DSM identifies *atypical anorexia* as a specific subtype of eating disorder.[38] This category describes a person who has all of the behavioral and physical symptoms of anorexia nervosa but is still at or above "normal" weight, usually because the starting weight was higher. Typically, these individuals have been praised and encouraged for their "success" at weight loss, when they are, in fact, quite sick. One study found an average of 13 years between onset of the illness and accurate diagnosis.[39] Once a diagnosis is made, quality treatment may be difficult to access because of unexamined weight bias among eating disorder treatment professionals.[40]

Weight Stigma Maintenance

Body shame flourishes in our world because profit and power depend on it.
—Sonya Renee Taylor, from *The Body Is Not an Apology*[41]

The weight loss industry generates enormous profits by promoting weight stigma. Sonya Renee Taylor, in her excellent book *The Body Is An Apology*, refers to this as the global Body-Shame Profit Complex.[42] Not only is there money to be made from diet products that do not work, but there is even more revenue in garments designed to squeeze the body into more acceptable shapes, clothing to hide "flaws," and replacement wardrobes for each episode of weight cycling. Food advertising successfully incorporates the moralizing tone of weight stigma by using such terms as "guilt-free" or "decadent." The pharmaceutical corporations profit from selling products, whether pills or lap-band devices. This body terrorism promotes self-hate while profiting from shame and bias.

The scientific research field, where there is some assumption of neutrality, is also saturated with anti-fat bias and stigmatizing discourses that endorse unexamined prejudices while persistently ignoring the lived perspectives of fat people. If scientists believe in the myths that weight is controllable and that weight loss always improves health, they are not going to be open to information that challenges their bias. Some researchers believe that encouraging positive body image, which is associated with improved self-care, is a problem because people *should* be dieting instead.[43]

Most literature about weight stigma focuses on the stigmatized target, the fat person, while ignoring the sources of the stigma, which are then invisible and unaccountable. Some of the research about weight stigma focuses on the ways it interferes with weight loss attempts, further reinforcing bias. Most research on weight stigma focuses on how it affects fat people, which implies that thinner people are not affected by it at all. It rarely addresses intersectionality. When research is funded by institutions or corporations that profit from weight stigma, the papers that actually get published will reflect the desired outcome; findings that contradict it will get buried. This contributes to public approval of discrimination toward fat people, even when it is openly hostile.

Weight stigma in research is largely unquestioned due to confirmation bias in researchers and editors. When I was taking a public health class, one of the assigned readings was a paper about conditions and behaviors related to morbidity and mortality. The authors used BMI as a measure of diet and exercise. It seems obvious, to me at least, that BMI is not a valid determination of either diet or level of physical activity, but this unexamined assumption was published in a prestigious medical journal, without question. In another example, an extremely well-designed study found that sustained weight loss in people with diabetes was not associated with improved health;[44] the paper about it was rejected by numerous journals because it contradicted the prevailing belief that weight loss should always be recommended as part of diabetes treatment.[45] At the same time, research funding is difficult to obtain if it is not couched in terms of "obesity prevention."[46] The scientific literature on weight and weight stigma is, in and of itself, a structural form of stigma.[47]

The medical profession also plays a role in maintaining weight stigma. In 2013, the American Medical Association defined obesity as a disease, when previously it had been considered a risk factor. This was in direct contradiction to the recommendations of its own Council on Science and Public Health, which had concluded that the designation was questionable and that the potential risks of defining obesity as a disease were greater than the benefits. The arguments in favor of such a change included increased funding for research and treatment. Counseling, medications, and surgeries for weight loss would be covered by insurance. Members of the AMA could make more money by treating obesity if it is considered a disease.

Critics of this decision point out the likelihood of increased stigma and focus on individual responsibility for change while neglecting more effective approaches, such as population-based interventions. They expressed concern that increased stigma would lead to poorer health behaviors and outcomes, and they recommended that the AMA reconsider its decision.[48] Weight becomes a moral issue when individuals are expected to try to become smaller for the benefit of the community, even as those selling weight loss products become richer.[49]

Meanwhile, those individuals who have invested enormous time, energy, and money in trying to maintain a lower body weight feel cheated when they are informed of the futility of their efforts. New information is often uncomfortable, especially when it exposes previously unacknowledged prejudice. At the same time, people who are preoccupied with body size have less time and energy to do other things that might be disruptive. Naomi Wolf, in her book *The Beauty Myth*, says, "A culture fixated on female thinness is not an obsession about female beauty, but an obsession about female obedience. Dieting is the most potent political sedative in women's history; a quietly mad population is a tractable one."[50]

The Role of Public Health

Interventions that are designed to change the health dynamics for groups and populations have sometimes been coercive. Decisions in the best interest of community health at times run counter to self-determination. One example that springs to mind is the recurring debate about raw versus pasteurized milk. Proponents of raw milk say that it has better nutritional value and that they should be allowed to acquire and consume it if they want. Laws requiring the pasteurization of commercially sold milk came about because of widespread illness and death, especially in children, as a result of diseases that raw milk carried. Are those laws coercive? Some people argue that they are. Most of us, however, are content to know that the milk we buy at the store is unquestionably safe for our children to consume.

We have already seen the evidence that a focus on behaviors is more likely to promote good health than a focus on weight loss, but many public health professionals, in both direct program delivery and in policy-making positions, are steeped in culturally endorsed weight bias. Anti-obesity efforts as part of public health initiatives contribute to weight stigma. Fat-shaming messages both encourage and condone discrimination.[51]

Public health programs usually focus on large groups, but anti-obesity efforts end up focusing on changing the body size of individuals. This focus on individual responsibility for health leads to prejudice, bias, stigma, and greater social surveillance of bodies. This increases the likelihood of an adipophobicogenic environment where people in fatter bodies are viewed with increasing disapproval. This weight-centered health paradigm is ineffective, harmful, and unethical.[52] Additional ethical concerns include masking discrimination and limiting freedom of choice while promoting the very stigma that is associated with adverse outcomes.[53]

The use of fear is controversial in the field of public health. Describing the awful effects of the flu as well as its potential to be deadly may influence a few more people to get flu shots, but at what cost? Fear creates and reinforces stigma, and it sometimes serves as a way to consolidate power by creating and disempowering marginalized groups. An argument can be made that public health marketing that deliberately exposes people to fear is a kind of deliberate trauma.[54]

Human rights and dignity are linked to individual and population vulnerability to disease. Generally, public health officials are operating from a place of power in the social hierarchy. Their programs are often aimed at marginalized populations, such as minority groups or people living in poverty. They have the ability to label differences as undesirable, thus stigmatizing them from a place of power.[55] They have an ethical responsibility to examine the uses of this power very carefully.

Numerous public health campaigns have used stigma and shame in the belief it is an effective way to change behavior. In the cases of drunk driving, smoking, and wearing seat belts, this method may have been effective. Weight, however, is not a behavior, and this approach is harmful. Stigma does not increase motivation to engage in healthier behaviors, nor does it lead to weight loss. Public health interventions need to be based on evidence of what works.[56]

Social Determinants of Health

The term *social determinants of health* refers to the conditions in which people live. They are shaped by money, power, and distribution of resources. They affect both health risks and outcomes. They include, among other things, such factors as adequate housing, safe neighborhoods, access to medical care, income, access to quality education, and safe working conditions.

According to the University of Wisconsin Population Health Institute, there are four main social determinants of population health. The physical environment, which includes the built environment and environmental quality, accounts for 10 percent. Socioeconomic factors, such as income, employment, education, community safety, and social support, account for another 40 percent. Access to and quality of health care comprises 20 percent, and health behaviors, such as diet, exercise, and use of tobacco or alcohol, only account for 30 percent. In other words, factors outside of individual behavior comprise 70 percent of social determinants of health.[57]

Socioeconomic status (SES) is a robust predictor of health, and a wealth of information exists to support that fact. Rich people are healthier than poor people. Kind-of-rich people are healthier than not-quite-so-rich people, and kind-of-poor people are healthier that really poor people. There is also a relationship between low social status and high body weight, especially for women in developed countries. Many factors influence this, and the interactions are complex.

The term *food insecurity* refers to the condition of being without reliable and sufficient access to food. During times of war or famine, entire populations may experience food insecurity, but the term commonly refers to situations in which there is not enough money, even though food is available for purchase. It is often a chronic condition. Food stamps are a social support program that is designed to make sure that families have enough to eat, but they are usually too meager to last the month.

Food insecurity is related to higher body weight. Critics wonder how someone can get fat if they do not get enough to eat, but there is a connection. Food deprivation, which is often experienced for the last few days of the month, when money and food stamps have run out, leads to compensatory overeating when food is available again, at the same time causing metabolic changes that promote weight gain. Food insecurity also increases stress and the hormone cortisol, which is associated with weight gain. In addition, those with fewer financial resources have a limited access to food variety and to safe physical activity. They may also have limited time for food preparation, relying on highly processed, energy-dense foods that stretch the budget.[58]

Financial inequities contribute to moralizing about food choices. People who have always had access to a plentiful variety of food underestimate the difficulties in feeding a family on food stamps or other limited resources. When middle-class food values are imposed on populations that are already marginalized by poverty, we are widening the divide between the haves and the have-nots.

Unexamined sexism plays into the pattern of blaming mothers more often than fathers. Even when the focus is on "parents," the interventions tend to be targeted at women. Programs that focus on providing more education and information about healthy eating and food preparation are often based on unrealistic views of the practical matters related to limited resources.

Meanwhile, mothers who are doing the best they can are held responsible for the fatness of their children.[59] The incorrect assumption that changing body size is simply a matter of improving intake and activity places the responsibility of children's size on the person who feeds them. The definition of a "good mother" is then based on having thin, healthy children. This unattainable goal undermines any sense of efficacy and competence in the parent, increasing feelings of shame and worthlessness. As Natalie Boero explains, "Evaluating the fitness of mothers based on the size of their children obscures larger structural issues of racism, economic inequality, fat phobia, and sexism, among others."[60]

When moral values of good and bad are placed on foods, they carry over to the people who consume them. However, the values themselves usually originate from a place of financial security and reflect additional unexamined assumptions. To read the articles and comments that appear regularly in various media, a common pastime for grocery shoppers is to criticize the choices they see in other carts when the purchases are being paid for with food stamps. The ability to buy fresh fruits and vegetables rather than snack cakes is a type of privilege. Anyone who has ever fed a child knows that children are reluctant to try new foods and will often flatly refuse to eat something they do not want. Advice about introducing children to new foods encourages repeated exposure over time. Parents who have limited money for food simply cannot afford to buy food that will be refused over and over.

Parents love their children and want to do what is best for them. Parents want to do things to make their children happy. Parents who have generous financial resources can treat their children with video game systems, violin lessons, soccer camp, athletic equipment, and vacations. Parents who are not sure that they can afford to pay the electric bill still want to give their children treats, even if all they can manage is a soda or a candy bar.

The relationship between higher body weight and lower SES has been a topic of much speculation. Many theories concentrate on how being poor makes people fatter, focusing on limited access to fresh fruits and vegetables, whole foods, and safe spaces for physical activity. In fact, there is reason to believe that the relationship also works the other way around: being fat makes people poorer through discrimination.

Employers hold stereotypical views about body weight because they are exposed to cultural bias, like anyone else. Multiple studies have shown that heavy people are less likely to be hired or promoted and more likely to be harshly disciplined or fired.[61] Lower employment opportunities, lower wages, less access to training, and inferior assignments lead to lower SES. This kind of discrimination is legal throughout most of the United States.

Body weight influences social mobility. Thin people from a lower class are more likely to be upwardly mobile, improving their SES, while fat people from wealthier backgrounds are more likely to move downward in terms of SES. Fatness is impoverishing. Stigma and discrimination prevent fat people from moving up the social ladder.[62]

Education is a consistent predictor of socioeconomic status, health, and well-being, yet large people are discriminated against at all levels of educational achievement, contributing to a significant and persistent wage gap. This is especially true for large women, who are less likely to start or finish college. They receive fewer offers to attend graduate school after in-person interviews when compared to women of average weight.[63]

American culture has an underlying historical foundation in the concept of meritocracy. This is the belief that people who are talented and deserving, who work hard, will rise to the top. This is the concept of "pulling yourself up by the bootstraps." In other words, self-determination combined with effort, willpower, and self-discipline will result in achievement and prosperity. When applied to body size, this results in fatness being seen as a failure of character, a moral defectiveness. A corollary of seeing fatness as a personal moral failure is that attempts at weight loss then indicate moral worth and responsibility, reinforcing harmful behavior. Virgie Tovar explains, "Dieting maps seamlessly onto the preexisting American narrative of failure and success as individual endeavors."[64]

Interventions to address weight concerns often take the form of education, because there is an assumption that people just do not know any better and can be taught to make better choices. Focusing on education is much easier than addressing social and economic disparities. This approach is racist and classist. It becomes a smokescreen for maintaining the social hierarchy which benefits the "experts."

The evidence is compelling. The best thing you can do for your health is to be rich. If you cannot be rich, at least do not be poor.

If SES is the primary predictor of health and well-being, then interventions designed to improve health must focus on improving opportunities and changing social policy. Focusing on individual responsibility distracts from social change. It relieves those in power from the accountability to change the systems that maintain inequity. Fat prejudice then becomes a subtle way to discriminate against poor people without being overtly racist or classist. Systemic problems cannot be solved through individualized solutions. Focusing on bodily outcomes obscures the discussion of other socio-politico-economic realities. We cannot solve social stigma through weight loss.

Dismissing obesity as a result of personal failure increases stigma and excuses discrimination, becoming justification for treating people badly. It piles shame and blame on those who are already struggling against enormous odds. It places responsibility squarely on the shoulders of those who have the least ability to enact change.

When physical, mental, and social pathologies are defined as defects in individual biology, social change is seen as no longer necessary. Institutionalized bias becomes an excuse for inaction regarding efforts to address disparities in the social determinants of health. Stigma has a fundamental influence on both individual and population health and needs to be addressed directly. If we truly want people to be healthier, individually and as a population, a focus on improving social determinants of health would be much more effective, even essential.

Social Change

Weight stigma causes serious problems at many levels and in many ways. How do we make it illegitimate and unacceptable? What can we do about it? We can perhaps do more than you think. Remember the Underpants Rule: you get to decide what you are willing to do, when, and how often.

If we focus on a *well-being* solution rather than a weight solution in our lives and in our conversations, we can open up to new ideas. When we accept body diversity instead of trying to eliminate differences, something shifts in us over time. When we engage in conversations about weight, health, nutrition, or food, we can look for a way to mention the social determinants of health; we can reframe stigma as discrimination rather than blame.

What you choose to do involves many variables. How comfortable are you about speaking up in one situation versus another? How safe are you if you argue with someone at work about a policy or plan? Are you able to risk a disruption in a relationship? What is your position in the world? Are you a person who makes decisions and policies for others? Who hears your words? What influence do you have?

Consider your privilege and how you can use it in a positive way. What can you challenge? A friend told me about being in a casual social situation when a man told a "fat joke." When she took offense and objected to it, he asked, "Why does it matter to you? You're not fat!" She responded, "I don't have to be black to object to racism, I don't have to be Jewish to object to anti-Semitism, I don't have to be gay to object to homophobia, and I don't have to be fat to know that your joke was mean-spirited."

If you have thin privilege or beauty privilege, you are more likely to be taken seriously if you speak up about stigma. At the same time, everyone has the right to object to the objectionable. If someone says something racist in a room full of white people, is it still racist? Of course it is. Would you say something about it? Probably. If someone says something objectionable that is based in weight stigma, can you react in the same way? Can you find a way to help someone think differently?

Those in positions of authority can be approached gently. Some years ago, when my children and I were taking tae kwon do, one of the instructors made some self-disparaging comments about his weight and his body in front of the whole class. I pulled him aside later and respectfully pointed out to him what an enormous influence he had on the kids in the room and how much more positive an influence he could be if he spoke about his own body with more kindness. He was very thoughtful because he had never considered it that way before. I never heard him speak meanly about his body again. Similarly, a friend recently posted a poignant letter online that she had written to her pastor. Acknowledging her own thin privilege, she explored all the ways that his self-directed fat jokes reinforced stigma and were potentially damaging to those who heard and respected his words.

Think ahead about what you might say when the situation presents itself. There is the all-purpose, "Why would you think it's okay to say that?" or "I realize you may not have thought of this, but do you realize that a comment like that contributes to weight stigma/body shaming?" A more pointed personal response might be, "When you say that, you let me know exactly how you feel about my body." Of course, it is always okay to say nothing at all. For more (often humorous) options, see Ragen Chastain's excellent book *Fat: The Owner's Manual*.[65]

Look around your workplace. Does the furniture accommodate people of size? If there is a waiting room, do the magazines on the table promote the thin ideal? If there is artwork, does it reflect diversity in body size? If there are brochures, do they include unexamined weight stigma? If you identify any concerns, is there someone in authority you can discuss it with? If you are the authority, change it! You can make the argument that if public spaces are supposed to be accessible to people in wheelchairs, why would you not have comfortable furniture for people of all sizes as well?

A tricky issue is wellness programs. While there are some approaches that consider diversity and social justice concerns, there are others that do not. If your employer or Human Resources Department is pushing a program that encourages dieting or otherwise promotes weight stigma, consider how to approach them (understanding that what you choose, including doing nothing, is entirely up to you, because Underpants Rule). To quote the incomparable Deb Burgard, "Show me the data!" Ask them to provide documentation that their program works in the long term and that it does not cause harm (because they will not be able to). If you need to support your own argument, start with the article "The Weight-Inclusive versus Weight-Normative Approach to Health: Evaluating the Evidence for Prioritizing Well-Being over Weight Loss."[66] This wonderful article is also useful if your doctor recommends weight loss for whatever ails you.

If you are in an educational setting, opportunities surround you. If you are a schoolteacher, watch for ways to intervene in conversations among the students to remind them that bodies come in all shapes and sizes and that everyone deserves to be treated with respect. Check to see if your school's antibullying resources include body size. If not, insist that it be added. Review the resources for health classes and see if they need revision. Look for ways to share information with other teachers and faculty. If you are a college professor, be creative about including new information. For instance, a class in statistics or research design could use one of the articles I have cited as a sample for study. If you are a student, ask questions or challenge information (within the etiquette of your classroom) if weight-stigmatizing concepts are taught. Consider choosing a related topic for research papers and provide lots of documentation to support it.

Other ideas include writing a letter to the editor of your local paper if it publishes articles or editorial cartoons that promote weight stigma or finding out if the local school system has a health and wellness committee and volunteer to be a part of it. If you belong to a group that regularly has speakers and presentations, suggest a Health At Every Size program. You might be able to find a local speaker at the website for the Association for Size Diversity and Health.

Sometimes opportunities unexpectedly present themselves. I recently stopped by my doctor's office to pick up something when a woman came by announcing an open house in the new outpatient surgery clinic "with cookies!" Of course, I walked down to check it out, and to be polite before claiming my cookie, I toured the suite. As I approached the snack table, the (thin) woman in charge asked whether I had any questions. "No," I said, "but I do have a comment. I am an eating disorder therapist. Your scale is out in the open in the hallway. Some people are traumatized by being weighed, especially in a nonprivate space like that." She was very thoughtful and agreed that a more secluded place might be found. It had not occurred to her before that it might be a problem, and she was open to the idea of doing it differently to improve patient care. Perhaps I made a difference, and all because I wanted cookie. (It was yummy.)

A social justice approach does not ask whether the glass is half empty or half full. Social justice asks, "Do you know that the glass is refillable? Who or what is stopping you from accessing the tap? What can we do about that?"

Healthism

According to Sonya Renee Taylor, "Health is not a state we owe the world. We are not less valuable, worthy, or loveable because we are not healthy."[67]

Health concerns have been and still are regularly used to justify stigma and discrimination by medical and public health professionals, and everyone else. The prevailing belief that health is strongly tied to weight is behind much of the rhetoric about the "need" for weight loss. I have been reviewing the evidence that weight stigma is damaging to individual and population health, in and of itself. A separate concern is how this framing may make people with chronic illnesses feel excluded. How can we expand this conversation to make sure that everyone feels included? Another question that deserves consideration involves whether the pursuit of health is always, or ever, the best focus. Each individual with the right of self-determination gets to decide how much priority to place on health. If someone chooses to eat poorly and avoid exercise, that is their right, just as choosing to bungee jump or swim in shark-infested waters is their right.

Many factors that affect our health are beyond our control, but underlying attitudes of healthism can cause unwarranted feelings of guilt and shame. One common example is the response that many people have to being diagnosed with diabetes. Referring to it as a "lifestyle disease" carries an implication that a person caused her own disease by not doing something right. I cannot count the number of times I have had someone in my office expressing great distress at having "brought this on myself," often after trying very hard to follow a healthy lifestyle. One young woman broke down in tears when telling me that her cat had been diagnosed with diabetes. "I'm a bad cat-mommy!"

This "blame the victim" mentality is racist and classist because it ignores the social determinants of health as well as the systemic effects of injustice. It reinforces a social hierarchy that assumes a superiority of healthy people and blames anyone who has the misfortune to be poor and sick for their situation. It ignores the effects of oppression as well as the roles of power in determining health.[68]

Healthism: This refers to a belief system that sees health as the property and responsibility of the individual. It assumes health is derived from correct body/mind management practises. It sees the pursuit of health in this way as a moral obligation, ranked above everything else, like world peace or being kind.

It ignores the impact of poverty, oppression, war, violence, luck, historical atrocities, abuse and the environment from traffic, pollution to clean water and nuclear contamination and so on. It protects the status quo, leads to victim blaming and privilege, increases health inequities and fosters internalized oppression.

Healthism judges people's human worth on the basis of their health, and often also on their degree of commitment to healthist beliefs and behaviours.[69]

Tugboats

When the task of effecting social change looms huge and overwhelming, I like to think of tugboats. Imagine an enormous ocean liner, steaming through the waves on the vast expanse of the sea. When that ship comes to shore, however, it cannot navigate the tight spaces of the port. At that point, the lowly, unflashy tugboats gather and persistently bump against it until, slowly, its direction changes. Usually the passengers on the ship do not even notice, but the vessel docks and then leaves again with the help of the humble tugboat.

We may not be able to change the world right now, but we can contribute to incremental changes that add up over time. We can all be a tugboat.

As John Pavlovitz says, "I don't speak to the bully to change the bully; I speak so those being bullied can hear."[70]

CHAPTER EIGHT

Going to the Doctor (and Other Adventures in Medical Care)

Weight stigma poses significant challenges to obtaining good medical care. It is difficult to put your well-being into the hands of someone who might shame you or may already have done so. Unfortunately, medical professionals are influenced by the same propaganda about the alleged benefits of weight loss as the rest of society.

Accessing adequate medical care in a timely manner is one more way that you give yourself a message about what you are worth. If you are sick or injured but persist in tolerating the discomfort, you are giving yourself a message that you are not worthy of good care. Knowing your rights and insisting on weight-neutral care at the doctor's office is a message that you have value, just the way you are.

I know, I know, easier said than done. You get to decide what you are willing to do (because Underpants Rule), but other people have been down this path and have come up with some ideas and strategies.

Linda Bacon's book *Health at Every Size* contains some sample letters and scripts to use when dealing with medical professionals, and there are additional resources on her website.[1] HAES-oriented websites and groups address this issue on a regular basis. Many people struggle with what to say.

The first step is to breathe and stay calm, if you possibly can. If you have difficulty advocating for yourself, is there someone who can go with you? It seems to be human nature that we can stand up for someone else better than we can for ourselves, so a friend or family member who understands your quest for weight-neutral care is a wonderful asset.

If you are dealing with a new provider, you have the option of calling or writing in advance to express your unwillingness to discuss weight loss. You can even provide some HAES-oriented information. If you are large, you can ask about whether their equipment will fit you.

Let's take this step-by-step. When filling out the paperwork, be honest about any eating disorder history or behaviors you may have. Questions about weight history may or may not represent weight bias. (Somewhere I remember reading about a woman who, when asked to list her lowest adult weight, answered, "When I was hospitalized for anorexia, so I don't know.") You can choose to write, "I do not want to discuss weight loss" at the top of the form.

The most dreaded part of going to the doctor is getting weighed. Almost everyone hates this part. Writing a number on the chart (or entering it in the computer) is built into the quality indicators that, supposedly, show that people are doing their jobs. They are required to document signs (something measurable by someone else, such as temperature or blood pressure) as well as symptoms (as experienced and reported by the patient, such as anxiety or pain), so they want to write down as many signs as they can. Being weighed, however, is considered a procedure, and procedures can be refused.

Most of the time, your weight has no bearing on your treatment. The main exception to this is congestive heart failure. If you have a condition or a treatment that is known to cause weight fluctuations, such as chemotherapy or thyroid imbalances, then monitoring weight may be necessary. If the doctor will be prescribing a medication that requires different dosages depending on size (something that happens more often in pediatric treatment than in adult treatment), weight is important; otherwise, it is rarely necessary. If you want to have your weight monitored when you go in for your yearly checkup, that is a valid choice. If, on the other hand, you avoid your checkup in fear of the scale, good self-care requires a better plan.

There are several options regarding the scale. You can simply say "No," or "Not today," or "I'd rather not." If the person who is checking you in insists or argues, you can ask for written documentation of a medical reason that it is needed. You can suggest that they write down "refused." If the computer will not go to the next screen, suggest a placeholder number, such a "001," because a computer does not get to override your self-care.

Dealing with the scale at the doctor's office is an ongoing topic of conversation among people with diagnosed eating disorders and the people who treat them. Treatment often involves relinquishing a focus on the numbers on the scale. Blind weights are done with the patient stepping on the scale backward and the treatment provider documenting the number without comment. This allows the assurance that weight is being monitored by a professional who will intervene in a therapeutically appropriate way if there is reason for concern. This works well until the individual has to go to a medical appointment. I have lost count of the number of stories I have heard from individuals who assertively state, "I am in treatment for an eating disorder; please don't say anything," as they get on the scale backward, only to have the nurse say, "Great! You are down/up 10 pounds!" or something equally problematic.

Lexi, a teenage girl in treatment with me for anorexia nervosa, also went to a pediatrician who specialized in eating disorder treatment. The weighing process was handled very well, as would be expected. However, the checkout person printed out and handed her a summary of the appointment that included her weight at the bottom. Lexi was able to discuss it with me, and I called the doctor so he could change the procedure. Many other offices would not have been able to even acknowledge the problem. Increasingly, medical offices use a health portal, which can be accessed online by the patient and usually includes information about weight and possibly distressing comments such as "obese." Clearly these systems were not designed with eating disorders in mind. There is no easy answer to this dilemma.

Stepping on the scale in a medical office can be traumatizing. If you have been harmed in the past, or think you could be harmed in the present, then it is good self-care to refuse. Being forced to weigh is like someone stealing your biological information without your consent and then possibly using it against you. You get to choose a different way to experience your body. If you educate someone along the way, that is nice, but not necessary. What works best for you?

Personally, I agree to be weighed at my yearly physical only. I have been refusing weights for years, if only to make a point. Most of the time, it is not a big deal, although I realize this reflects a certain amount of thin privilege that I still have. However, once I went to an Urgent Care clinic that was in the same system as my primary care physician. I was too sick to have the energy to argue with the very insistent nurse, so I got on the scale wearing my coat, hat, and boots while carrying my purse and book. Interestingly, no one ever commented on my weight fluctuation!

Once you get past the dreaded scale moment, there you are in the office. If the process so far has been distressing, try to take some deep breaths before your blood pressure is taken. If the number is higher than usual, ask for it to be taken again in a few minutes. Large people are especially at risk with this. Medical professionals may assume that your blood pressure is high based on their own weight bias and may be more likely to question a low reading than a high one. A cuff that is too small will also result in an inaccurately high reading. One way to advocate for yourself as a large person is to ask for a larger cuff. Sizing for cuffs is not standardized, but they generally come in adult, large adult, and adult thigh. Adults who are underweight sometimes need a pediatric cuff for accuracy. The tag on the cuff may state what size arm it best fits. Some individuals have gone so far as to buy their own larger cuff to take with them to appointments if they know the office does not have one. Monitoring your own pressure at home with a wrist cuff and document-ing the results provides more information, but wrist cuffs may not be as accurate as arm cuffs.

If you feel that your doctor is being too quick to prescribe blood pressure medication based on your size and one reading, you can ask to have it taken again. There is a documented medical phenomenon called *white coat hyper-tension*, which is seen in people who get anxious the moment the medical professional walks into the room. Having your own record of your blood pressure taken at home over time is a good defense for this. Accurate read-ings are especially important during pregnancy, when an inaccurate high blood pressure reading can indicate a medical emergency where none exists.

Now we get to the really tricky part, dealing with the doctor. The doctor is the expert in medicine; you are the expert in you. If the doctor cannot work with you in a partnership, that is her problem, not yours. Your problem is being able to access appropriate treatment anyway. If the doctor comments on your weight or starts talking about weight loss, your response could include something like, "I'd like to focus on the reason I am here, which is my sore throat/rash/compound fracture," or "I am not interested in discuss-ing my weight today," or "What would you prescribe for a thinner person with this problem?" Depending on how assertive you are feeling, you could say, "You have not asked me about my exercise or how I eat. Would you like to know?" Another response to persistent focus on weight loss recommenda-tions is, "Show me the data! Can you show me at least three peer-reviewed articles about the approach you are recommending that document sustained significant weight loss for the majority of people who try it over at least three years?" If the recommendation is for weight loss surgery, ask, "Do you have documentation that it results in significant weight loss at least five years later without major medical complications or death?" or even "Do you get a finan-cial incentive for referrals?"

Remember, you have a right to informed consent. In fact, using the phrase "informed consent" might change the conversation. Ask, "Have you told me about all the possible side effects or negative outcomes associated with what you are recommending?" If you feel that the doctor is ignoring your com-plaints and you have a specific concern that is not being addressed, it may be useful to state, "I want you to document in my chart that you are not order-ing the test I am asking for and why." This is moderately confrontational, but if you are concerned that something serious is going on, it may get you the test that you need. This is also a good time to have someone with you who can act as an advocate.

If you have a bad experience at a medical appointment, how do you process that? Speaking up in the moment is scary and overwhelming. Writing a letter later is also an option. You may be doing someone a favor by educating them about a point of view they have not considered. You may be doing a favor for future patients. Primarily, though, writing a letter afterward gives you a chance to express your feelings and let go of shame for yourself, regardless of what reaction the medical staff has.

Arguing with your doctor is not without risk, and you get to decide what to do in any specific circumstance. Sometimes you may need to find a new doctor. Everyone deserves to have a trusting, mutually respectful relationship with a primary care physician. With specialists, you may have less choice but also less interaction. Interactions with surgeons, for instance, mostly happen when we are already anesthetized. Psychiatrists, on the other hand, may or may not be understanding about your need to accept your body just as it is, but you might need one to manage your medication anyway.

The magic of the Internet makes it easier to find HAES-friendly medical practitioners. The Association for Size Diversity and Health has an extensive list of HAES-informed professionals on their website. Online body-acceptance groups often share recommendations as well as information about fat-phobic practitioners to avoid. As with most things, it is easier to find resources in a big city than in outlying rural areas. Finding someone good is better than finding someone convenient. Keep looking until you find a good fit, if you can.

The belief that anyone can change treatment providers because they are unhappy assumes a certain amount of privilege. Availability may be limited by insurance, ability to pay, or geographic distance. Sometimes people get stuck with doctors that they do not like, particularly specialists, because there is no other option. If that happens, try and remember that the weight stigma is the problem—you are not the problem—and consider the source. Use your own filter and do your best to disregard weight shaming.

Clarissa is a large woman with diabetes who began seeing me a couple of years ago for chronic depression. We have discussed self-care in some detail, especially how her unreliable patterns of adequately nourishing her body affect her mood and self-esteem. She recently told me about an appointment with her endocrinologist, a man known to focus on weight loss. She took a friend with her as an advocate. When the doctor began scolding her, basically saying, "You brought these problems on yourself with your lifestyle," she and her friend were both able to argue with him. He apparently had not read the report in the chart of her recent hospitalization involving an adverse reaction to medication that was still causing the abnormal readings in her blood work that he was blaming on her weight.

Instead of accepting the shame, she was able to speak up for herself, with the help of her friend. She told me, "If that had happened a couple of years

ago, it would have sent me into a long spiral of major depression!" We discussed the possibility of writing a letter, not to necessarily change the doctor
but to assert her own feelings. Fortunately, she has the option of changing
doctors and plans to do so.

Regrettably, this idea of "You brought this on yourself" is not uncommon,
especially regarding diabetes. The amount of guilt and shame experienced
by people with this diagnosis is damaging in and of itself, yet an individual
person has very limited control over many health risks, including diabetes.
Most health factors have a large genetic component, which, of course, we
cannot control. While we have some control over health behaviors, such as
exercise, the ability to engage in healthy behaviors is influenced by socioeconomic factors. We should not have to "earn" good medical care. Everyone has
the right to expect respectful treatment from medical professionals, regardless of size, age, gender, socioeconomic status, or health behaviors.

If you feel you have been treated badly or disrespectfully at the doctor's
office because of your body size, remember that the problem is not located in
your body, it is in the bias of the medical professional.

CHAPTER NINE

But What about the Children?

Concern about the well-being of children is hardwired into adults; without it, the human race would not have survived. Concern for children is not exclusively the domain of parents; if we are concerned about the toxic effects of diet culture, we are concerned about the ways it affects not just ourselves and the people in our lives, but everyone. This chapter is for anyone who has children, nieces, nephews, friends, and coworkers with children, neighbors, or other contact with young people.

Parents, understandably, want their children to have good lives. If parents or other caregivers have suffered from unkind behavior because of their weight, it is natural for them to want to avoid that for the children they love. Unfortunately, this often takes the form of focusing on the child's weight and trying to avoid fatness or weight gain at any cost.

It is altogether understandable that parents who were bullied, harassed, or mistreated as children because of their weight would want to spare their children the same experience. Unfortunately, focusing on weight only perpetuates the problem. Just like with adults, learning to value the variety of sizes and shapes that occur naturally in the population while discussing healthy behaviors that benefit everyone leads to better outcomes with youngsters, too.

Everything that is true regarding adults about food, eating, health, weight, and well-being is also true about children, often more so. We have no reliable way to make fat children thinner, and attempting to do so causes more problems. Yet we continue to see much focus on the "childhood obesity epidemic."

There is no evidence that this generation of children will live shorter lives than their parents because of obesity, but the headline sells advertising and harmful weight loss programs. The trend of increasing life expectancy in the United States does not stop the hype, which can be downright terrifying. I have seen headlines about "The first generation of children to not outlive their parents," which taps into every parent's worst fear. This idea is a perfect example of what Jon Robison calls the "cockroach effect."[1] It is an idea that originated in an offhand remark by a researcher to a reporter, who took it out of context and ran with it. The researcher tried to withdraw the comment, but it spread like cockroaches and is now an infestation, impossible to eradicate. There is no evidence to support the idea that obesity will shorten the lives of our children, but the concept continues to plague us.[2]

In fact, the documentation that links increased body weight to increased life expectancy has been growing for more than a century. At the same time, the evidence for an "obesity epidemic" caused by too much junk food and screen time among young people is vague, contradictory, and far from definite.[3]

A common misconception is that fat children are unhappy because they are fat. In fact, anxiety, body dissatisfaction, and loneliness are more related to experiences of weight stigma, such as disrespectful or exclusionary behaviors by other children, rather than body size.[4] Bullying is the problem, not body size.

Bullies are people who reinforce their own sense of worth by belittling someone else. There are many ways to respond to bullying, but trying to change your body to appease the bully is unlikely to have a good outcome. If a child of color is bullied because of the color of his skin, we do not encourage him to try to be more white. If a child is bullied because of a physical disability, we do not tell her to try to be more able-bodied. Nor do we tell a short child to try to be taller. Why, then, is weight-based bullying often met with recommendations to lose weight? It goes back to the myths we talked about earlier, the pervasive mistaken belief that weight is something that we can control. Bullying is a behavior that is difficult to address, but blaming the victim does not change the bully. As adults, there are many ways we can support children who are distressed without focusing on weight change. We must teach them that it is the bullies who are wrong.

Children learn best by example. Parents and other caregivers who have been bullied about their weight may have their own issues with body image, self-worth, and shame. They may still be buying into the idea that there is something wrong with them that they should change. This deprives their children from the in-group support that safety in group membership provides, including stigma buffering, psychological resources, and self-worth (see also chapter 7).[5] Imagine a child in a household of a family that is marginalized by race, ethnicity, or religion. The adults do not bemoan their identity and try to change it. Instead, they identify and talk about the social inequalities that affect them, take comfort in belonging to a group, and build resilience in one another. They may discuss interventions for social change. They may express anger at those who mistreat them. They may address security concerns and ways to safely deal with the larger society. They teach their children that they have value, just the way they are.

Social support, especially when it emphasizes available resources, helps children cope with stigma. Stress-buffering support from nurturing parents lessens mental and physical risks associated with adverse experiences with discrimination such as bullying. When parents warmly help children by teaching about stigma and promoting group identity, then self-esteem, behavior, and coping abilities improve. A sense of safety and belonging decreases vigilance and increases a sense of worth.[6] Being able to do this requires that parents recognize and address their own internalized weight stigma.

Health Concerns

The alleged "obesity epidemic" among children has led to pervasive fear mongering about the health risks to our children. This is particularly difficult to navigate as a parent because caregivers are blamed when children do not fall into a "normal" weight range. One exceptionally difficult example is the inflated concern of the relative risk of developing diabetes, as it is commonly considered a lifestyle disease caused by overeating and underexercising. The threat of a diabetes diagnosis is then used to justify bullying people in larger bodies. Type 2 diabetes is more complicated than that, and it is rarely seen in children. Eating disorders are more common. Estimates vary, depending on definition: one source documents eating disorders as affecting from 8.6 percent to 13.2 percent of people under the age of 20.[7] A more commonly quoted number is 10–15 percent.[8] Only 0.26 percent of children under the age of 20 have type 2 diabetes, and only 7 percent of that 0.26 percent are under the age of 10.[9] That means that children under the age of 20 are about 34 times more likely to develop an eating disorder than type 2 diabetes, while those younger than 10 are about 430 times more likely. Given that anorexia nervosa has the highest mortality rate of any psychiatric diagnosis,[10] telling parents that their children will get diabetes because of their weight is a particularly hazardous type of fear mongering.

Putting children on a diet (or lifestyle change or any other approach that has weight loss as a goal) is dangerous and destructive. The behavior of dieting is a risk factor for both eating disorders and increased weight. Dieting in childhood or adolescence predicts a slower metabolism, weight gain, and obsession with food. Putting a child on a diet teaches her that her body is not acceptable, that she is not acceptable, and that her body cannot be trusted. Childhood dieting usually results in a lifelong battle with oneself, with resulting shame and low self-esteem.

Food restriction in childhood creates food insecurity and hunger, resulting in a chronic fear of going hungry. Just as we have seen with adults, this can lead to binge eating or secretive eating. Restricted intake may also result in inadequate nutrition, which interferes with growth. Some children, especially boys, need to get plump before they get tall. A well-meaning parent or pediatrician who tries to prevent the child from becoming "too fat" may actually stunt his growth.

Children who are labeled as "too fat" (which is clearly implied when a child is put on a diet) are more likely to be labeled "obese" 10 years later, regardless of their actual weight in childhood.[11] Body dissatisfaction in adolescents increases risk of weight gain and poorer health.[12] Parental focus on weight status and food restriction are associated with decreased self-evaluation in girls as young as five.[13] Parents who restrict what their children eat may inadvertently be contributing to weight gain and psychological harm.[14] When parents focus on weight, children do not learn to be thinner; they learn to be dissatisfied with their bodies.[15]

The focus on "childhood obesity" paradoxically puts thin children at risk, too. All children benefit from eating a wide variety of tasty, nutritious foods and engaging in enjoyable physical activity. Naturally thin children (and their parents) may internalize the idea that they can survive on highly processed snack foods and spend all of their time being sedentary in front of a screen because they mistakenly think that their very thinness indicates that they are healthy. Those same children may then experience a growth spurt and panic about the accompanying weight gain, responding with unhealthy weight control measures. Other naturally thin children can internalize the weight stigma they are exposed to in the world and at home and develop a debilitating fear of gaining weight, accompanied by disordered eating.

The incidence of eating disorders has increased at the same time that the focus on "preventing childhood obesity" has increased. In a society that considers watching one's weight as a moral obligation, the culture of dieting is normalized, and anorexia nervosa is framed as a normal consequence. Weight stigma, in the form of perceived pressure to be thin as well as an internalized thin ideal, is significantly elevated in youngsters who develop eating disorders before the onset of the illness.[16] Eating disorders are usually thought of as affecting rich, white teenage girls, but they are increasing in other populations. Between 1999 and 2006, the number of children under the age of 12 who were hospitalized for eating disorders increased by 119 percent.[17] Eating disorders are not about vanity or attention seeking, and they are the psychiatric disorder with the highest mortality rate. Eating disorders almost always start as weight loss diets or attempts to "eat healthy." Body dissatisfaction and dieting behaviors are related to a threefold increase in disordered eating and weight gain.[18]

Food restriction in childhood creates food insecurity, hunger, and a fear of being hungry. This disrupts the child's natural ability to tune into bodily cues, especially regarding appetite. Limiting specific foods, such as sugar or sweets, teaches a child that such foods are more desirable and can lead to overconsumption when those foods are available in another setting.

Meanwhile, unexamined weight stigma strongly influences the current discourse about weight and its effect on the well-being of young people. This raises several important concerns. When authority figures, such as parents, teachers, coaches, and doctors, routinely berate young people about their weight in the context of expressing concern for the target's health, these comments may be experienced as vicious personal attacks. Abusive fat talk is considered acceptable, even required. Subjects then perceive themselves as "biologically flawed, morally irresponsible or unworthy, or aesthetically unappealing, or some combination of the three."[19] This results in serious consequences:

> The nationwide campaign to banish obesity and make people healthy seems to be producing anything but thinness, health, and happiness. . . . Far from producing thin, fit, happy young people, the war on fat is producing a generation of tormented selves, heart-rending levels of socioemotional suffering, and disordered bodily practices that pose dangers to their health.[20]

Building Resilience

What can we do with our children instead? We cannot prevent our children from encountering body shaming in the world, but we can give them an underpinning of body positivity and self-directed eating. We can discourage dieting behavior, discourage conversations about weight, promote positive body image, encourage enjoyable family meals, encourage a healthy attitude about eating and physical activity, and be open to talking about negative experiences associated with weight.[21] Shifting the focus from dieting and weight control measures to healthful eating and physical activity will improve outcomes for both obesity and eating disorders.[22] It is important to remember that all children benefit from these interventions, not just the ones who are larger or who have been identified as at risk for body image concerns.

What works with adults works with children: legalizing and neutralizing all foods while avoiding judgmental labels (e.g., "bad foods"); accepting all bodies as having worth; praising characteristics and abilities instead of appearance; supporting awareness of physical sensations and eating from an internal locus of control; engaging in fun physical activity and play; and acknowledging that food is a source of pleasure and enjoyment.

Children learn more from example than from instruction. If they hear you making disparaging comments about your own body or about other people's bodies, that is what they learn. When they hear conversations about "feeling fat" or attempts to lose weight, they learn that being fat is terrible and to be avoided at all costs. If they see weight-based bullying that is ignored by grownups, they learn that this is acceptable. Weight stigma is learned.

If your child hears you say disparaging things about people with large bodies, she may be afraid that you will stop loving her if she gains weight. If you treat people of all sizes with respect, your child learns that human worth is not contingent on body size.

Notice how you talk about your own body. If you find yourself saying negative things, think about what effect that has on the child listening to you. If you struggle with your own body image, can you start by making neutral or positive comments, even if you do not altogether feel comfortable with it? It does not have to be about appearance: "I like the way this fits me because I can move freely in it," or "This dress may not be new, but I still love the way I feel in it," or "I'm glad I have big strong thighs to help me lift and carry you!"

It is possible to promote healthy eating without endorsing diet culture and mentality. Talk about how our bodies need a variety of nutrients and where they come from. Explain how we need protein for muscles and vitamins for eyesight. Avoid talking about calories, but be prepared to respond if the subject arises. Remember, calories are a measure of energy, and energy is what we need to learn, play, and live our lives. Try and adjust the information to the developmental stage of the child and avoid overloading young children with more than they can understand. As much as possible, provide children with a wide variety of foods to choose from and allow them some autonomy in their choices.

Children are born with a strong internal locus of control about hunger and eating. Newborns know when they are hungry and when they are full. Limiting what and how much a child eats interferes with the ability to recognize hunger and fullness, an effect that can last a very long time and lead to disordered eating in the future. Ask judgment-neutral questions to build conscious awareness of their bodies and their hunger. A question like, "Are you hungry or are you just bored?" carries an implication that it is not okay to ask for something to eat. "Haven't you had enough?" undermines the child's natural ability to determine satiety. However, if the child later complains of being too full, it is an opportunity to say, "Remember this the next time you eat that food. Can you check in with your stomach to see when it is almost full so this doesn't happen again?"

When you encounter the ever-present "good food/bad food" message, take the opportunity to talk about it. Emphasize that all foods have a place in a normal diet that incorporates a variety of choices. Messages about "healthy foods" with children are more likely to increase anxiety than to improve health. Even the old standard of "You have to eat your vegetables if you want dessert" reinforces an artificial hierarchy, making dessert more valuable and vegetables less appealing. Obviously, if a child has an allergy or other medical reason to restrict certain foods, that must be addressed as well, but it can be done in the context of "What is right for your body" rather than "bad food."

Involving children in food preparation has many possible good results. Cooking together is often an enjoyable activity for adults and can be just as fun for youngsters if the tasks are age appropriate. Children are more likely to try new foods if they have helped fix them. Food is not just about fueling our bodies; it is about creativity, pleasure, and enjoyment. Planning, preparing, and partaking in a delicious meal is a wonderful way to learn. Plus, being able to cook for oneself is a valuable life skill that all children deserve to learn.

Physical activity offers many ways to be a role model. Be mindful of what you do and also how you talk about it. When children see adults engaging in movement for fun, relaxation, and enjoyment, they are more likely to do the same. If children observe adults complaining about how much they dislike exercise and commenting that they only do it to lose weight, they develop a different attitude. Talk about how good it feels to move, how certain activities build strength and stamina, and how exercise can result in new friendships.

Consider activities to do together. Many martial arts schools welcome families and participants of all ages. Taking tae kwon do classes with the children in your life provides a new way to bond and interact while working out. Yoga studios are another option for age-inclusive classes. Roller skating and ice-skating are additional alternatives. Of course, walking, hiking, swimming, and informal sports can be done together. If your child plays an organized sport, such as soccer, check into training to be a referee. Everyone can exercise while having fun together.

Pay attention to how adults compliment children. It may be easier to comment on appearance, "Oh, you look so pretty!" but think about how that reinforces the idea that value is based on appearance. Instead, try to focus on function or abilities. "I love watching you run down the field; you are so swift!" or "I could tell you worked really hard on that," or "I enjoyed your company; it was so much more fun because you were with me." Children have so many positive characteristics besides how they look. Be creative and comment on intelligence, perseverance, loyalty, dependability, good judgment, friendliness, compassion, honesty, creativity, perceptiveness, or sense of humor. What do you wish you had been more valued for when you were young? Can you find a child who needs that kind of feedback and offer it?

Similarly, if a child asks, "Am I fat?" the response is often, "No, sweetheart, you are beautiful," which reinforces the idea that appearance is all-important. Other options include, "Your body is growing exactly the way it is supposed to," or "Remember how we have talked about trusting your body to know how much to eat? Your body knows what it needs to grow." Keep in mind that teenagers are still growing, too. They may not be getting taller, but their bones, muscles, and organs are still developing and need nutrition. This continues into adulthood. After all, we would not expect members of a high school football team to be the size of college football players, and vice versa.

Talking with children about the unrealistic images on television, in movies and over social media teaches them to be more observant and thoughtful. Media literacy is the ability to realistically evaluate what we see in movies, television, magazines, and online. Until about the age of seven, children cannot tell the difference between advertisements and programming. Conversations about television can be especially helpful in developing discernment about ads, attitudes, and product placement. Even small children can see when characters in a show are being mean to one another and can talk about what makes that not okay. Engaging older children in conversations about advertising is also fruitful. Ask questions like, "Is this ad trying to make us feel a certain way? What emotion is it encouraging? Is it trying to make me ashamed so I will buy the product?" Point out product placement, such as diet sodas in the background in shows with only very thin people. Ask, "Why do you suppose that they chose to run this ad on this particular show?" Observe that most people we see on television or in movies are predominantly white, young, thin, and able-bodied and do not represent the general population. Talk about what it might be like to see a wider variety of both adults and children on the screen. Reinforce the idea that there is no one right way to have a body.

The American Academy of Pediatrics recognizes that weight stigma affects children in negative ways and needs to be addressed. The recommendations for their members include focusing on healthy, sustainable habits, such as physical activity and eating a variety of foods, rather than on weight, while discouraging dieting behavior such as skipping meals or using diet pills; promoting positive body image and avoiding using body dissatisfaction as a reason for dieting; encouraging more family meals; encouraging conversation about healthy behaviors rather than weight; and inquiring about bullying and addressing ways to deal with it.[23]

The World

No matter how well you deal with these issues at home, sooner or later your child will go out into the world. Unless you are willing to homeschool on an isolated outpost with no Internet or television, your child will encounter weight stigma. Unfortunately, one of the biggest sources of stigmatizing messages will probably be the school.

If you are committed to a weight-judgment-free approach to life and child-rearing, you will most likely encounter some conflict with the educational system. You get to choose how to respond (because Underpants Rule). Sometimes a friendly email to the educator involved can open the possibility of further communication. A good place to start is a reminder that we all want what is best for the children. Gently providing more information about how a certain policy or procedure may, in fact, cause harm initiates a new conversation. If you are questioning a policy, ask for data that shows that it is safe and effective, because many interventions are only based on what someone thinks is a "good idea."

Some elementary schools have a person in the lunchroom to police what the children are eating and in what order. There may be a policy about what can be included in lunches packed at home. Ask whether there is an opt-out possibility, which can encourage a different way of thinking. Sending a note or email along the lines of, "At our house, we practice weight-neutral, self-regulated eating. I want my children to be able to eat as much or as little of the items in their lunches as they choose and in whatever order they choose." Keep in mind that there is a big difference between rules that are focused on weight manipulation and rules that protect a child with severe allergies.

School-based interventions that focus on weight, even extensive, well-funded programs, make little difference in children's weights or metabolic measures.[24] Unintended consequences include increasing stigma among children and adults, overlooking lifestyle risks in thin children, and promoting concerns about appropriate eating in all children.

Considerable evidence confirms that weight stigma exists in school settings and that it causes harm. "Anti-obesity" interventions are linked to increased social stigma, especially for heavier girls, while "obesity rates" are unchanged.[25] "Obesity prevention" programs are often implemented without evidence to show that they are helpful or that they avoid inadvertent harm. The risks of BMI screening in schools include increased weight stigma, increased body dissatisfaction and disordered eating, decreased self-esteem, and increased likelihood of parents putting children on diets.[26] Parental awareness of a child's status as "overweight" does not necessarily translate into helpful behaviors and may increase unhelpful behaviors.[27] Appearance-related teasing in the home is related to body dissatisfaction, disordered eating, depression, and low self-esteem.[28]

Many school districts have mandated health classes, usually in middle or high school. These are often taught by teachers who have minimal understanding of the health risks inherent in promoting weight stigma, and they may themselves have problems with eating or body image. If you can, ask to see the curriculum. The nutrition component may have a strong emphasis on weight loss. The eating disorder component may be triggering for youngsters who are struggling with their own eating issues. Ask if you can have your child excused from those sessions. Some teachers show movies such as *Super Size Me* without realizing the stigmatizing messages they contain. Some cases of eating disorders have been traced to health classes that focus on the dangers of weight gain. Some information is inappropriate for youngsters who, developmentally, have black-and-white reasoning. Trying to eat "healthy" or "clean" can quickly become extreme.

An excellent resource to share with school personnel is "Guidelines for Childhood Obesity Prevention Programs" found on the website for the

Academy for Eating Disorders.[29] It includes a short but comprehensive over-view of the ways that interventions focused on weight cause harm rather than good. The specific and useful suggestions offer ways to focus instead on promoting health for all children, acknowledging the social determinants of health, promoting self-esteem and respect for body diversity, offering sugges-tions for using weight-neutral language, addressing bullying, and much more.

Additional resources can be found at the websites for Katja Rowell, at the Feeding Doctor (thefeedingdoctor.com), and Ellyn Satter, at the Ellyn Satter Institute (https://www.ellynsatterinstitute.org/).

Bullying

Sooner or later, most children (and many adults) will experience some form of bullying. Hopefully, a child who is being bullied has available adults to confide in and can access adequate support. Remember, the problem is the bully's behavior and not the characteristics of the one being bullied.

Attitudes about bullying have changed over time, but there is still support among some people for the idea that kids who are being bullied just need to toughen up or fight back. Bullying is not character building; it is a form of abuse. It is a pattern of behavior that is repeated and intentional, often with a goal of building social power. It reinforces the us-versus-them mentality, which encourages individuals to side with the winner and shun the loser.

At some level, bullying is based in a lack of empathy. Caring about other people's feelings is something that children learn over time. Toddlers do not have the capacity to imagine or value the feelings of another. Depending on the child's developmental stage, unkind behavior may represent an inten-tional desire to hurt or be simple thoughtlessness. However, intention is not the same as outcome. "I was only teasing" or "I didn't mean anything by it" are not acceptable reasons to let the behavior go unchallenged. If a child (or any-one, for that matter) says, "This made me feel sad/scared/upset/distressed," those feelings need to be acknowledged, even if the hurt was unintentional.

When a child comes from a background that encourages empathy and values body diversity, the child will be less likely to engage in bullying behavior and more likely to be resilient if targeted by a bully, but that may not be enough. Pay attention if the child has sudden changes in mood or begins to avoid certain places or activities; gently encourage some conversa-tion about it. When talking about difficult topics, remember to first focus on reinforcing the behavior of talking. Save problem-solving for later. Expres-sions of outrage or suggestions for fixing the problem are likely to end the flow of information. Find out as much as you can about what has been hap-pening first. Before offering suggestions, ask, "What have you tried?"

Sometimes a bully will say, "You better not tell anyone!" Many child safety programs stress teaching children that if someone says, "Don't tell your mother!" the first thing to do is tell your mother (unless it involves birthday presents). Hopefully, the children in your life know that they can tell you anything, especially when they have been told not to tell. If the situation is serious enough to warrant action on your part, start by getting as many details as you can and write them down. Documentation may not be necessary, but it is better to have it and not need it than to need it and not have it.

Each situation is different and will require different responses. If the bullying happens at school or on the bus, find out what the school's policy is and what resources are available there. If the policy does not include weight, body size, and appearance as protected categories, suggest that they be added. Point out that children deserve to be protected from bullies and that they may be targeted because someone thinks they are too short/too tall/too thin/too heavy/too light/too dark. Children with a higher weight are uniquely vulnerable, though, because even adults may believe that body shaming will motivate them to lose weight. If you encounter this, demand to see proof: "Show me the data! Show me proof that shaming children results in better health and behavior! Show me the research that proves that this approach does not cause harm!"

Usually the best person to start with is the child's teacher. If that is not enough, it may be necessary to talk with the principal, the superintendent, or the school board. It is helpful to start those conversations with something like, "We all want the best possible learning environment for all of our children. How can we work together to address this barrier?"

Weight-based bullying can also happen in churches, youth clubs, sports teams, or other places where children gather. Other settings are less likely to have written policies about dealing with it, but they hopefully still have concerned adults to address the issue.

Unfortunately, one of the common places that size-based bullying happens is within the family, where it is potentially more damaging that elsewhere.[30] For the sake of the children, find ways to set limits with family members, including aunts, uncles, grandparents, stepparents, cousins, or siblings about what kind of talk is not acceptable. Be firm. Again, "I'm only teasing" is not an acceptable excuse. "I'm just trying to toughen her up" is even worse. If necessary, explain to your child in private that the person is misguided. Be a role model: if an adult is body shaming another adult, intervene, even if it is only to change the subject. Consider seeking out the target of the meanness later to acknowledge what happened and express support.

Antibullying resources include ideas for empowering children by discussing options and role-playing. Children (and adults) are less likely to be bullied if they have a confident stance and voice. It may help to practice these things, but be cautious about putting more responsibility on the child than is appropriate or feasible. Practice some responses that are not argumentative, insulting, or demeaning. "Why would you think it's okay to say that?" is a favorite of mine. "Have a nice day" or another neutral response might take the bully off guard. Remind the child that walking away is always an option.

The child's safety is paramount. Physical bullying is assault and may need to be reported to law enforcement or child protection.

I have been very aware as I write this section that many of these suggestions (and most of the reading I have done on the topic) assume a certain amount of privilege, and I want to acknowledge that. Not all parents and guardians have the time and flexibility to engage with school systems to address problems. Protecting a child from a weight-bigoted family member is risky if you are financially dependent on that person. Single parents who are working two or three jobs to make ends meet will struggle to even get to parent-teacher conferences. Most parents are trying to do the best they can to care for their children. Just as the problem of bullying resides in the bully, not the target, the problem of limited resources lies in the system, not you.

CHAPTER TEN

What Now?

If you have made it this far through the book, hopefully you have some clear ideas about changes that you can make to improve your quality of life. Now, where do we go from here?

Fortunately, there are many more resources available to help you continue your body-love journey. Unfortunately, there are a lot of sources that look good but are not. Trust your own filter and intuition to evaluate them. There are countless books and articles about what we should be doing in the pursuit of health and happiness, and there is even more information online. No one can evaluate all of them, but I will offer some ideas for where to begin. First, let's talk about what to look for in reading material.

When evaluating a book, if there is any focus at all on weight loss or avoidance of "eating too much" or an assumption that weight loss is a valuable goal, be very careful. It does not mean that all the information is wrong, but it is distorted by the lens of weight loss. Pay attention to how you feel when you read. If you experience any sense of shame, guilt, or failure, put it down. If you have thoughts along the lines of, "It wouldn't hurt me to lose a few pounds," put it down. It may be valuable to sit with the feelings for a bit and see whether you can learn anything. If you realize that the book is causing bad body thoughts, abandon it. (If it is from the library, return it. If you own it, consider using it for garden mulch.)

A disclaimer: I love to read, and I love to recommend books. Through the years, I have recommended many books to clients, and I have listened to their feedback. I have learned that not everyone loves the same books I love, or they do not respond to them in the same way. I have tried to incorporate that knowledge into this list.

Some of My Favorite Books

Beauty Sick: How the Cultural Obsession with Appearance Hurts Girls and Women, by
Renee Engeln, PhD. If you are interested in cultural pressures and how they

affect body image and quality of life, this is a great place to start. The information is particularly helpful for men who want to understand more about the way women experience life in our society. Not everyone is this good at talking about one's own research while still being an interesting read.

The Body Is Not an Apology: The Power of Radical Self-Love, by Sonya Renee Taylor. We can push back against the systems of oppression that make money by making us insecure and heal our own injuries in the process. The book's cover is a guaranteed conversation starter!

Binge Eating Disorder: The Journey to Recovery and Beyond, by Amy Pershing and Chevese Turner. The authors offer an innovative understanding that binge eating may be a reasonable coping response for surviving trauma, thus offering new approaches for treatment.

Body of Truth: How Science, History, and Culture Drive Our Obsession with Weight—And What We Can Do about It, by Harriet Brown. This is a thorough, but not overly technical, review of the science of weight and health along with ideas and suggestions for change. This is often the first book I suggest to anyone who wants to know more about this topic.

Fat-Talk Nation: The Human Costs of America's War on Fat, by Susan Greenhalgh. Based on qualitative research using essays written by college students, Dr. Greenhalgh shares poignant, often heartrending, accounts of the way individuals are affected by well-meaning comments about weight and bodies. Again, this author is interesting when writing about her own research.

Health at Every Size: The Surprising Truth about Your Weight, by Linda Bacon. If you really want the science, this is the book to read. It is brilliant, but some folks find it kind of technical. It is truly a paradigm-shifting publication.

Body Respect: What Conventional Health Books Get Wrong, Leave Out, and Just Plain Fail to Understand, by Linda Bacon and Lucy Aphramor. The authors examine the science of weight and health through a lens of social justice.

You Have the Right to Remain Fat, by Virgie Tovar. This is an intriguing mix of memoir and astute observations of cultural pressures, with an emphasis on the racial and cultural biases beneath fat phobia.

Fat: The Owner's Manual, by Ragen Chastain. Yes, this is the same Ragen Chastain who formulated the Underpants Rule. Subtitled "Navigating a thin-obsessed world with your health, happiness and sense of humor intact," it is filled with humorous and helpful ways to negotiate life in a fat-phobic world.

Fat!So? by Marilyn Wann. This book provides activism, information, and guidance. Plus, if you remember how to do those flippy-page books from your childhood, there is the wonderful dancing fat lady in the corner.

The Angry Chef's Guide to Spotting Bullsh*t in the World of Food: Bad Science and the Truth about Healthy Eating, by Anthony Warner, a chef with a biochemistry degree. He thoroughly and humorously debunks diet fads, from alkaline to paleo to detoxing to "clean eating."

Real Gorgeous, by Kaz Cooke. Written for teenagers, this is a fun read that is full of cartoons, imaginative graphs, and helpful suggestions.

Killer Fat: Media, Medicine, and Morals in the American "Obesity Epidemic," by Natalie Boero. This offers a fascinating overview of various approaches to weight loss and how they reinforce social control.

Overcoming Overeating and *When Women Stop Hating Their Bodies*, by Jane Hirschmann and Carol Munter. These are considered "classics" in the field. When I recommend *When Women Stop Hating Their Bodies* to married women, I suggest that they warn their husbands that they are likely to be cranky while reading it, as it examines what the culture has taught us about our bodies that is harmful.

Beyond a Shadow of a Diet: The Therapist's Guide to Treating Compulsive Eating Disorders and *The Diet Survivor's Handbook: 60 Lessons in Eating, Acceptance and Self-Care*, by Judith Matz and Ellen Frankel. These useful publications are practical, applicable, and easy to read. Besides, *Beyond a Shadow of a Diet* just has to be the best book title ever!

Big Fat Lies, by Glenn Gaesser. This is the second best book title ever. The author provides more science with an emphasis on health and fitness.

The Dieter's Dilemma, by William Bennett and Joel Gurin. First published in 1982, this book introduces the concept of the *set point*. Unfortunately, it is out of print, but it is well worth tracking down at a library or used bookstore.

Women Afraid to Eat and *Children and Teens Afraid to Eat*, by Frances Berg. The author examines how dieting and a preoccupation with slenderness compromise adequate nutrition and how that affects other aspects of one's life.

The Spirit and Science of Holistic Health: More Than Broccoli, Jogging, and Bottled Water . . . More Than Yoga, Herbs, and Meditation, by Jon Robison and Karen Carrier. Health At Every Size (HAES) concepts are explored through the lens of the biomedical model and the myth of scientific objectivity.

Child of Mine: Feeding with Love and Good Sense, by Ellyn Satter. I also recommend everything else written by Ellyn Satter. She is the go-to person for any and all questions about children and eating.

Helping Your Child with Extreme Picky Eating: A Step-by-Step Guide to Overcoming Selective Eating, Food Aversions and Feeding Disorders, by Katja Rowell, "the Feeding Doctor," and Jenny McGlothlin, a speech and feeding therapist, offers evidence-based, practical solutions to family food struggles.

For resources about exercise, especially for people who have been sedentary and are considering more activity, I recommend *Great Shape*, by Pat Lyons and Deb Burgard, *The Fat Chick Works Out!* by Jeanette DePatie, and *The Unapologetic Fat Girl's Guide to Exercise and Other Incendiary Acts*, by Hanne Blank.

Resources that focus more on history, culture, and society include the following:

Unbearable Weight: Feminism, Western Culture, and the Body, by Susan Bordo, explores the links between Western cultures, mind/body dichotomy, and the cult of thinness.

Losing It: False Hopes and Fat Profits in the Diet Industry, by Laura Fraser, addresses the history and impact of the dieting industry.

Fat Blame: How the War on Obesity Victimizes Women and Children, by April Michelle Herndon. This is a thoughtful examination of cultural aspects of weight stigma and how they affect those who are already marginalized by class, race, age, and gender.

The Obesity Myth, by Paul Campos. Media misinformation and body-based prejudice is explained from a lawyer's perspective.

Beauty Bound and *Body Love*, by Rita Freedman. These classics provide a valuable understanding of culture and body image.

The Body Project, by Joan Jacobs Brumberg. The author examines historical attitudes about women's bodies.

Fat Shame: Stigma and the Fat Body in America, by Amy Erdman Farrell. Drawing on a wide array of sources, this volume offers an historical analysis of multiple cultural issues regarding body size.

Catching Fire: How Cooking Made Us Human, by Richard Wrangham, a biological anthropologist. I particularly enjoy his evolution-based assumption that weight gain is always good and weight loss is always bad!

The Great Starvation Experiment: The Heroic Men Who Starved So That Millions Could Live, by Todd Tucker. This is a fascinating insight into the people and the process of the classic starvation experiment, much easier and more fun to read than Keys's *Biology of Human Starvation*, the original study.

Revolution at the Table: The Transformation of the American Diet, by Harvey Levenstein. Cultural eating patterns in the United States in the last two centuries have an intriguing history.

Healthy Bodies: Teaching Kids What They Need to Know, by Kathy J. Kater, is a curriculum for addressing body image, eating, fitness, and weight concerns in educational settings, and it contains great background information.

Dispensing with the Truth: The Victims, the Drug Companies, and the Dramatic Story behind the Battle over Fen-Phen, by Alicia Mundy, and *Tipping the Scales of Justice*, by Sondra Solovay, JD, address some of the legal issues around weight stigma.

Women and Shame, by Brene Brown, is not specifically about eating or weight, but it does provide valuable insight into how the powerful emotion of shame limits our lives.

Fat Politics: The Real Story behind America's Obesity Epidemic, by J. Eric Oliver, argues that our concern with obesity is more about profit and social prejudice than is it about health.

The Fat Studies Reader, edited by Esther Rothblum and Sondra Solovay, is a wonderful collection of chapters written by many highly qualified experts in the field, ranging from health and social inequality to popular culture and embodiment.

What's Wrong with Fat? by Abigail Saguy, a cultural sociologist, explores the many ways that fatness is defined in current society and the many problems with the current understanding.

The Politics of Size: Perspectives from the Fat Acceptance Movement, edited by Ragen Chastain, is a two-volume collection of chapters by different authors (including me). It covers a wide range of topics, such as activism, physical and mental health, education, and athletics.

When you find a book that resonates with you, consider sharing it with important people in your life. My client Sarah recently talked with me about her husband's request to understand her eating disorder better. The thought of trying to explain her difficulties to her very logical, methodical husband made her quite anxious. She is currently reading *Beauty Sick*, so we came up with idea that she read it out loud to him while he is driving on their upcoming road trip. She felt more confident when she thought about using someone else's words as a starting place for discussion.

Internet resources change so quickly that I cannot begin to list them all. More information can certainly be found by checking out the websites of any of the authors listed here and by exploring their links as well. Websites for the Renfrew Center and the Association for Size Diversity and Health are also good places to start. Many other good resources exist on the Internet, but many more pages filled with dieting mentality and shame are lurking out there. Again, use your own filter to evaluate them.

When Reading Is Not Enough: Finding More Help

Sometimes reading and acquiring new information is enough to bring about change and healing. At other times, it only reveals the tip of an iceberg that requires more specialized care. Reestablishing adequate nutrition and normalizing eating may expose other issues that the pursuit of weight loss has disguised. Working with a weight-neutral, weight-inclusive therapist or dietician may be necessary. If nutrition is seriously compromised, it is difficult to address psychological issues, because brain function is affected. Occasionally, a higher level of care, such as residential or inpatient, is required. This is generally recognized in people with a diagnosis of anorexia nervosa because of their obvious low weight. However, it may also be true for those with atypical anorexia, bulimia, or binge eating, as the undernutrition that results from the behavior of undereating can affect anyone at any body size. Ideally, care involves a treatment team that includes a physician, a dietician, a therapist, and others, but that may only be available in large cities or at big medical centers.

Professional qualifications can be confusing. Licensing laws vary from state to state, but their focus is on protecting the public from unqualified practitioners. If a treatment professional is licensed, that is documentation of a minimum of training and expertise in that particular field. For instance, a *registered dietician* has completed specialized training, usually a minimum of a four-year bachelor's degree (and often a two-year master's degree), plus supervised practice and passed an exam. The term *nutritionist* means different things to different people who use it, and it may be used by registered dieticians as well as people with other training. A *counselor* is a person who has a master's degree in counseling plus supervised experience and has passed an exam. Counselors also participate in ongoing continuing education. A *social worker* is similar to a counselor, except with a degree in social work. A *licensed psychologist* usually has a doctoral degree in psychology and may have specialized training in assessment and evaluation.

A licensed professional may or may not have preparation for treating those with eating and body image concerns. Various types of "healers" with an assortment of qualifications can set themselves up in practice, but they are not regulated by any official group. Keep this in mind when looking for additional treatment.

Changing ingrained body shame and disordered relationships with food is challenging. Finding support is sometimes just as challenging. Professional therapists, counselors, psychologists, and dieticians are exposed to the same propaganda as the rest of us, so use caution when selecting one if you decide that is what you want to do. Counseling can be very helpful, even essential, when overcoming body image and eating issues, especially if you feel you are not making progress on your own. If you are able to reestablish nutrition and normalize your eating on your own, your dieting mind-set may have been effectively distracting you from other emotional issues in your life. Healing your relationship with food may uncover old unresolved concerns that will be difficult to sort out by yourself.

The first step is finding the right person. Most of my clients find me through an online listing, but keep in mind that not everyone is listed there, for various reasons. (For instance, there is website that lists "eating disorder therapists" that charges a hefty fee for the listing, so you will not find me on it.) Sometimes you can find leads simply by asking friends or your medical providers. It is worth the time and effort to find the right fit for you.

Here are some questions to start with: "Are you taking new patients?"; "Do you accept my insurance?" (if you are planning to use it); and "What are your hours?" (if you are limited in your own availability). If the answer to the first three questions is no, then it wastes everyone's time to ask anything else. "Do you treat adults with eating issues?" might be the next question, as some therapists only treat children or people with substance abuse issues, or they have some other limitations on their work. If so, ask whether they can suggest someone else.

Most therapists are willing to answer some questions on the phone about what they do. Answers to "Do you practice from a Health At Every Size perspective?" or "What is your philosophy for treating body image/weight/eating problems?" should give you a sense of their approach. If they mention weight loss as a goal or imply that emotional problems cause weight gain, or something similar, say, "Thank you," and move on. There is no point in going into details about your own history before you establish that this is a person you want to see.

Therapy is a collaboration. The therapist is an expert in counseling, while you are an expert in you. If you do not understand something, ask for more explanation. If you do not like the direction the therapist is going, say so. If you feel the process is moving too slowly, or going too fast, say that too. Your feedback and participation are essential and valuable. Accessing appropriate treatment is another message you give yourself about your own worth.

CHAPTER ELEVEN

Final Thoughts

Take care of your body. It's the only place you have to live.[1]

What if, tomorrow, everyone woke up happy with their body's appearance? How would the world change? If I had a genie in a bottle, that would be my first wish. Who knows what would be left to wish for if that happened?

Of course, it will not happen just like that. Change happens slowly for individuals and even more slowly for society. At the same time, individual efforts at change do matter, and they add up over time. What changes can you make? What changes are you willing to try?

I know it is not simple, and it will be easy to get discouraged. Ask yourself, "How many more resources and how much time and energy am I willing to invest in hating my body? What will I have if I stop? How much of my energy and cognitive resources am I wasting on monitoring my body and my intake? What else could I be doing with that time, energy, and money? How many ways might my life improve?"

Can you think of one thing that you would do differently if you loved your body exactly as it is right now? Is it possible to do that?

Our quality of life is influenced by countless factors, many of which we cannot control. We can control how we treat ourselves, how we talk to ourselves, and how we value ourselves. You deserve to live your best life right now, in the body you have, to the best of your ability. You deserve to make your own choices about where you invest your time, energy, and money. You deserve to decide for yourself. I hope I have given you some ideas for how to do that.

Your body is valuable exactly as it is right now. Any other message is prejudice.

Live large! Live loud! Live well!

Namaste.

Notes

Preface

1. Terry Pratchett, *Going Postal* (London: Doubleday, 2004), 311.
2. William Bennett and Joel Gurin, *The Dieter's Dilemma: Eating Less and Weighing More* (New York: Basic Books, 1982).

Chapter 1: Where Are We, and How Did We Get Here?

1. American Psychiatric Association, *Diagnostic and Statistical Manual of Mental Disorders*, 5th ed. (Washington, DC: American Psychiatric Association, 2013).
2. American Psychiatric Association, *Diagnostic and Statistical Manual of Mental Disorders*, 3rd ed., revised (Washington, DC: American Psychiatric Association, 1987).
3. American Psychiatric Association, *Diagnostic and Statistical Manual of Mental Disorders*, 5th ed.
4. Rita Freedman, *Bodylove: Learning to Like Our Looks and Ourselves : A Practical Guide for Women* (Carlsbad, CA: Gürze Books, 2002), 29.
5. Marilyn Wann, *FAT!SO? : Because You Don't Have to Apologize for Your Size* (Berkeley, CA: Ten Speed Press, 1998).
6. American Psychiatric Association, *Diagnostic and Statistical Manual of Mental Disorders*, 5th ed.
7. Deb Burgard, personal communication, n.d.
8. Nancy LeTourneau, "What the $60 Billion Weight Loss Industry Doesn't Want You to Know," *Washington Monthly*, May 2, 2016, https://washingtonmonthly.com/2016/05/02/what-the-60-billion-weight-loss-industry-doesnt-want-you-to-know/.

Chapter 2: The Science of Weight and Health

1. Nancy LeTourneau, "What the $60 Billion Weight Loss Industry Doesn't Want You to Know," *Washington Monthly*, May 2, 2016, https://washingtonmonthly

.com/2016/05/02/what-the-60-billion-weight-loss-industry-doesnt-want-you-to -know.

2. Alison Fildes et al., "Probability of an Obese Person Attaining Normal Body Weight: Cohort Study Using Electronic Health Records," *American Journal of Public Health* 105, no. 9 (September 2015): e54–e59.

3. Linda Bacon, *Health at Every Size: The Surprising Truth about Your Weight* (Dallas: BenBella Books, 2008), 148.

4. Randy Dotinga, "The Average Americans' Weight Change since the 1980s Is Startling," CBS News, August 3, 2016, https://www.cbsnews.com/news /americans-weight-gain-since-1980s-startling.

5. J. Eric Oliver, "The Politics of Pathology: How Obesity Became an Epidemic Disease," *Perspectives in Biology and Medicine* 49, no. 4 (2006): 611–627.

6. Esther Rothblum, "Slim Chance for Permanent Weight Loss," *Archives of Scientific Psychology* 6 (2018): 63–69.

7. William Bennett and Joel Gurin, *The Dieter's Dilemma: Eating Less and Weighing More* (New York: Basic Books, 1982).

8. A. J. Stunkard et al., "An Adoption Study of Human Obesity," *New England Journal of Medicine* 314, no. 4 (January 23, 1986): 193–198.

9. E. Sims, "Studies in Human Hyperphagia," in *Treatment and Management of Obesity*, ed. George A. Bray and John E. Bethune (Hagerstown, MD: Medical Dept., Harper & Row, 1974), 28–44.

10. Ann E. Macpherson-Sánchez, "Integrating Fundamental Concepts of Obesity and Eating Disorders: Implications for the Obesity Epidemic," *American Journal of Public Health* 105, no. 4 (April 2015): e71–e85.

11. Andrea Bombak, "Obesity, Health at Every Size, and Public Health Policy," *American Journal of Public Health* 104, no. 2 (February 2014): e60–e67.

12. Harriet Brown, *Body of Truth: How Science, History, and Culture Drive Our Obsession with Weight—And What We Can Do about It* (Boston, MA: Da Capo Lifelong Books, 2015).

13. Paul Campos, *The Obesity Myth: Why America's Obsessions with Weight Is Hazardous to Your Health* (New York: Gotham, 2005).

14. David M. Garner and Susan C. Wooley, "Confronting the Failure of Behavioral and Dietary Treatments for Obesity," *Clinical Psychology Review* 11, no. 6 (1991): 729–780.

15. R. L. Leibel, M. Rosenbaum, and J. Hirsch, "Changes in Energy Expenditure Resulting from Altered Body Weight," *New England Journal of Medicine* 332, no. 10 (March 9, 1995): 621–628.

16. Traci Mann, *Secrets from the Eating Lab* (New York: HarperCollins, 2015).

17. Traci Mann, A. Janet Tomiyama, and Andrew Ward, "Promoting Public Health in the Context of the 'Obesity Epidemic': False Starts and Promising New Directions," *Perspectives on Psychological Science: A Journal of the Association for Psychological Science* 10, no. 6 (November 2015): 706–710.

18. Jon Robison and Karen Carrier, *The Spirit and Science of Holistic Health: More Than Broccoli, Jogging, and Bottled Water . . . More Than Yoga, Herbs, and Meditation* (Bloomington, IN: AuthorHouse, 2004).

19. A. Stunkard and M. McLaren-Hume, "The Results of Treatment for Obesity: A Review of the Literature and Report of a Series," *Archives of Internal Medicine* 103, no. 1 (January 1959): 79–85.

20. F. Grodstein et al., "Three-Year Follow-Up of Participants in a Commercial Weight Loss Program: Can You Keep It Off?," *Archives of Internal Medicine* 156, no. 12 (June 24, 1996): 1302–1306.

21. Tracy L. Tylka et al., "The Weight-Inclusive versus Weight-Normative Approach to Health: Evaluating the Evidence for Prioritizing Well-Being over Weight Loss," *Journal of Obesity* (2014): 1–18.

22. Orland W. Wooley and Susan C. Wooley, "The Beverly Hills Eating Disorder: The Mass Marketing of Anorexia Nervosa," *International Journal of Eating Disorders* 1, no. 3 (1982): 57–69.

23. Linda Bacon and Lucy Aphramor, "Weight Science: Evaluating the Evidence for a Paradigm Shift," *Nutrition Journal* 10, no. 1 (January 24, 2011): 1–13.

24. L. Bacon et al., "Low Bone Mass in Premenopausal Chronic Dieting Obese Women," *European Journal of Clinical Nutrition* 58, no. 6 (June 2004): 966–971.

25. Kathy J. Kater, "Why 'Obesity Prevention' Is Making Us Fatter, More Poorly Nourished, and Less Fit—The Need for a New Paradigm for Weight," BodyImageHealth.org, 2010, https://www.sizediversityandhealth.org/images/uploaded/Kater%20-%20White%20Paper,%20pdf.pdf.

26. Traci Mann et al., "Medicare's Search for Effective Obesity Treatments: Diets Are Not the Answer," *American Psychologist* 62, no. 3 (April 2007): 220–233.

27. Dianne Neumark-Sztainer et al., "Obesity, Disordered Eating, and Eating Disorders in a Longitudinal Study of Adolescents: How Do Dieters Fare 5 Years Later?," *Journal of the American Dietetic Association* 106, no. 4 (April 2006): 559–568.

28. Adam Gilden Tsai and Thomas A. Wadden, "Systematic Review: An Evaluation of Major Commercial Weight Loss Programs in the United States," *Annals of Internal Medicine* 142, no. 1 (January 4, 2005): 56–66.

29. Stunkard and McLaren-Hume, "The Results of Treatment for Obesity."

30. Wooley and Wooley, "The Beverly Hills Eating Disorder."

31. Garner and Wooley, "Confronting the Failure of Behavioral and Dietary Treatments for Obesity."

32. Leibel, Rosenbaum, and Hirsch, "Changes in Energy Expenditure Resulting from Altered Body Weight."

33. Christopher N. Ochner et al., "Treating Obesity Seriously: When Recommendations for Lifestyle Change Confront Biological Adaptations," *Lancet Diabetes & Endocrinology* 3, no. 4 (April 1, 2015): 232–234.

34. Garner and Wooley, "Confronting the Failure of Behavioral and Dietary Treatments for Obesity."

35. Leibel, Rosenbaum, and Hirsch, "Changes in Energy Expenditure Resulting from Altered Body Weight."

36. Macpherson-Sánchez, "Integrating Fundamental Concepts of Obesity and Eating Disorders."

37. Peter Muennig et al., "I Think Therefore I Am: Perceived Ideal Weight as a Determinant of Health," *American Journal of Public Health* 98, no. 3 (March 2008): 501–506.

38. Mann, Tomiyama, and Ward, "Promoting Public Health in the Context of the 'Obesity Epidemic.'"

39. Rachel P. Wildman et al., "The Obese without Cardiometabolic Risk Factor Clustering and the Normal Weight with Cardiometabolic Risk Factor Clustering: Prevalence and Correlates of 2 Phenotypes among the US Population (NHANES 1999–2004)," *Archives of Internal Medicine* 168, no. 15 (August 11, 2008): 1617–1624.

40. Paul Ernsberger, "Does Social Class Explain the Connection between Weight and Health?," in *The Fat Studies Reader*, ed. Esther Rothblum and Sondra Solovay (New York: NYU Press, 2009), 25–36.

41. Muennig et al., "I Think Therefore I Am."

42. Katherine M. Flegal et al., "Association of All-Cause Mortality with Overweight and Obesity Using Standard Body Mass Index Categories: A Systematic Review and Meta-Analysis," *JAMA* 309, no. 1 (January 2, 2013): 71–82.

43. Bombak, "Obesity, Health at Every Size, and Public Health Policy."

44. Lily O'Hara and Jane Gregg, "The War on Obesity: A Social Determinant of Health," *Health Promotion Journal of Australia: Official Journal of Australian Association of Health Promotion Professionals* 17, no. 3 (December 2006): 260–263.

45. Jacqueline Shaw and Marika Tiggemann, "Dieting and Working Memory: Preoccupying Cognitions and the Role of the Articulatory Control Process," *British Journal of Health Psychology* 9, Pt 2 (May 2004): 175–185.

46. A. Janet Tomiyama et al., "Low Calorie Dieting Increases Cortisol," *Psychosomatic Medicine* 72, no. 4 (May 2010): 357–364.

47. A. G. Dulloo et al., "How Dieting Makes the Lean Fatter: From a Perspective of Body Composition Autoregulation through Adipostats and Proteinstats Awaiting Discovery," *Obesity Reviews: An Official Journal of the International Association for the Study of Obesity* 16, Suppl. 1 (February 2015): 25–35.

48. Bacon and Aphramor, "Weight Science."

49. Peter Muennig, "The Body Politic: The Relationship between Stigma and Obesity-Associated Disease," *BMC Public Health* 8 (April 21, 2008): 128.

50. Abigail Saguy, *What's Wrong with Fat?: The War on Obesity and Its Collateral Damage* (New York: Oxford University Press, 2013).

51. K. Becofsky et al., "A Prospective Study of Fitness, Fatness, and Depressive Symptoms," *American Journal of Epidemiology* 181, no. 5 (2015): 311–320.

52. Katri Räikkönen, Karen A. Matthews, and Lewis H. Kuller, "The Relationship between Psychological Risk Attributes and the Metabolic Syndrome in Healthy Women: Antecedent or Consequence?," *Metabolism: Clinical and Experimental* 51, no. 12 (December 2002): 1573–1577.

53. M. D. Wirth et al., "Metabolic Syndrome and Discrepancy between Actual and Self-Identified Good Weight: Aerobics Center Longitudinal Study," *Body Image* 13 (March 2015): 28–32.

54. Bacon and Aphramor, "Weight Science."

55. Muennig, "The Body Politic."

56. Saguy, *What's Wrong with Fat?*

57. Sripal Bangalore et al., "Body-Weight Fluctuations and Outcomes in Coronary Disease," *New England Journal of Medicine* 376, no. 14 (April 6, 2017): 1332–1340.

58. A. Janet Tomiyama, Britt Ahlstrom, and Traci Mann, "Long-Term Effects of Dieting: Is Weight Loss Related to Health?," *Social and Personality Psychology Compass* 7, no. 12 (2013): 861–877.

59. Deb Burgard, personal communication, 2017.

60. Lucy Aphramor, "The Impact of a Weight-Centred Treatment Approach on Women's Health and Health-Seeking Behaviours," *Journal of Critical Dietetics* 1, no. 2 (2012): 3–12.

61. Richard D. deShazo, John E. Hall, and Leigh Baldwin Skipworth, "Obesity Bias, Medical Technology, and the Hormonal Hypothesis: Should We Stop Demonizing Fat People?," *American Journal of Medicine* 128, no. 5 (May 2015): 456–460.

62. Rebecca M. Puhl and Kelly D. Brownell, "Confronting and Coping with Weight Stigma: An Investigation of Overweight and Obese Adults," *Obesity* (Silver Spring, MD) 14, no. 10 (October 2006): 1802–1815.

63. Cat Pause, "Die Another Day: The Obstacles Facing Fat People in Accessing Quality Healthcare," *Narrative Inquiry in Bioethics* 4, no. 2 (2014): 135–141.

64. Marilyn Wann, *FAT!SO?: Because You Don't Have to Apologize for Your Size* (Berkeley, CA: Ten Speed Press, 1998).

65. N. K. Amy et al., "Barriers to Routine Gynecological Cancer Screening for White and African-American Obese Women," *International Journal of Obesity* 30, no. 1 (2006): 147–155.

66. Linda Bacon et al., "Size Acceptance and Intuitive Eating Improve Health for Obese, Female Chronic Dieters," *Journal of the American Dietetic Association* 105, no. 6 (June 2005): 929–936.

67. Bacon and Aphramor, "Weight Science."

68. Emily Dollar, Margit Berman, and Anna M. Adachi-Mejia, "Do No Harm: Moving beyond Weight Loss to Emphasize Physical Activity at Every Size," *Preventing Chronic Disease* 14 (2017): E34.

69. Eric M. Matheson, Dana E. King, and Charles J. Everett, "Healthy Lifestyle Habits and Mortality in Overweight and Obese Individuals," *Journal of the American Board of Family Medicine* 25, no. 1 (February 2012): 9–15.

70. Tylka et al., "The Weight-Inclusive versus Weight-Normative Approach to Health."

71. A. Keys et al., *The Biology of Human Starvation*, 2 vols. (Oxford, England: University of Minnesota Press, 1950).

72. Todd Tucker, *The Great Starvation Experiment: The Heroic Men Who Starved So That Millions Could Live* (Minneapolis, MN: Simon & Schuster, Inc., 2006).

73. Sims, "Studies in Human Hyperphagia."

74. Bennett and Gurin, *The Dieter's Dilemma*, 19–20.

75. O. G. Edholm et al., "The Energy Expenditure and Food Intake of Individual Men," *British Journal of Nutrition* 9, no. 3 (1955): 286–300.

76. Sarah E. Domoff et al., "The Effects of Reality Television on Weight Bias: An Examination of *The Biggest Loser*," *Obesity* (Silver Spring, MD) 20, no. 5 (May 2012): 993–998.

77. Jina H. Yoo, "No Clear Winner: Effects of *The Biggest Loser* on the Stigmatization of Obese Persons," *Health Communication* 28, no. 3 (2013): 294–303.

78. Kathrin Karsay and Desirée Schmuck, "'Weak, Sad, and Lazy Fatties': Adolescents' Explicit and Implicit Weight Bias Following Exposure to Weight Loss Reality TV Shows," *Media Psychology* 22, no. 1 (January 2, 2019): 60–81.

79. Erin Fothergill et al., "Persistent Metabolic Adaptation 6 Years after 'The Biggest Loser' Competition," *Obesity* 24, no. 8 (2016): 1612–1619.

80. James Fell, "'It's a Miracle No One Has Died Yet': *The Biggest Loser* Returns, Despite Critics' Warnings," *Guardian*, January 4, 2016, https://www.theguardian.com/tv-and-radio/2016/jan/04/the-biggest-loser-returns-despite-critics-warnings.

81. Domoff et al., "The Effects of Reality Television on Weight Bias."

82. Brown, *Body of Truth*.

83. Mann, Tomiyama, and Ward, "Promoting Public Health in the Context of the 'Obesity Epidemic.'"

84. R. Puhl, J. L. Peterson, and J. Luedicke, "Fighting Obesity or Obese Persons? Public Perceptions of Obesity-Related Health Messages," *International Journal of Obesity* 37, no. 6 (June 2013): 774–782.

85. Lisa Rosenthal et al., "Weight- and Race-Based Bullying: Health Associations among Urban Adolescents," *Journal of Health Psychology* 20, no. 4 (April 2015): 401–412.

86. A. Janet Tomiyama and Traci Mann, "If Shaming Reduced Obesity, There Would Be No Fat People," *Hastings Center Report* 43, no. 3 (June 2013): 4–5; discussion 9–10.

87. Bacon et al., "Size Acceptance and Intuitive Eating Improve Health for Obese, Female Chronic Dieters."

88. Christine E. Blake et al., "Adults with Greater Weight Satisfaction Report More Positive Health Behaviors and Have Better Health Status Regardless of BMI," *Journal of Obesity* 2013, Article ID 291371 (2013): 13 pages.

89. Marla E. Eisenberg, Jerica M. Berge, and Dianne Neumark-Sztainer, "Dieting and Encouragement to Diet by Significant Others: Associations with Disordered Eating in Young Adults," *American Journal of Health Promotion* 27, no. 6 (August 2013): 370–377.

90. Kathy J. Kater, John Rohwer, and Karen Londre, "Evaluation of an Upper Elementary School Program to Prevent Body Image, Eating, and Weight Concerns," *Journal of School Health* 72, no. 5 (May 2002): 199–204.

91. Amy M. Kelly et al., "Adolescent Girls with High Body Satisfaction: Who Are They and What Can They Teach Us?," *Journal of Adolescent Health: Official Publication of the Society for Adolescent Medicine* 37, no. 5 (November 2005): 391–396.

92. Dianne Neumark-Sztainer, "Preventing Obesity and Eating Disorders in Adolescents: What Can Health Care Providers Do?," *Journal of Adolescent Health: Official Publication of the Society for Adolescent Medicine* 44, no. 3 (March 2009): 206–213.

93. Dianne Neumark-Sztainer et al., "Does Body Satisfaction Matter? Five-Year Longitudinal Associations between Body Satisfaction and Health Behaviors in Adolescent Females and Males," *Journal of Adolescent Health: Official Publication of the Society for Adolescent Medicine* 39, no. 2 (August 2006): 244–251.

94. Neumark-Sztainer et al., "Obesity, Disordered Eating, and Eating Disorders in a Longitudinal Study of Adolescents."

95. David Benton, "The Plausibility of Sugar Addiction and Its Role in Obesity and Eating Disorders," *Clinical Nutrition* (Edinburgh, Scotland) 29, no. 3 (June 2010): 288–303.

96. Rebecca L. W. Corwin and John E. Hayes, "Are Sugars Addictive? Perspectives for Practitioners," in *Fructose, High Fructose Corn Syrup, Sucrose and Health*, ed. James M. Rippe, Nutrition and Health Series (New York: Springer New York, 2014): 199–215.

97. James M. Rippe and Theodore J. Angelopoulos, "Sugars and Health Controversies: What Does the Science Say?," *Advances in Nutrition* 6, no. 4 (July 1, 2015): 493S–503S.

98. Hisham Ziauddeen, Sadaf Farooqi, and Paul Fletcher, "Obesity and the Brain: How Convincing Is the Addiction Model?," *Nature Reviews Neuroscience* 13, no. 4 (2012): 279–286.

99. Jon Robison, "A Little Nutrition Sanity—Sugar: The Other White Powder—Rhetoric vs. Reality," LinkedIn, August 18, 2015, https://www.linkedin.com /pulse/little-nutrition-sanity-sugar-other-white-powder-rhetoric-jon-robison.

100. Angela Meadows, Laurence J. Nolan, and Suzanne Higgs, "Self-Perceived Food Addiction: Prevalence, Predictors, and Prognosis," *Appetite* 114 (July 2017): 282–298.

101. Ibid.

102. David Salsburg, *The Lady Tasting Tea: How Statistics Revolutionized Science in the Twentieth Century* (New York: Holt Paperbacks, 2002), 51.

103. Alicia Mundy, *Dispensing with the Truth: The Victims, the Drug Companies, and the Dramatic Story behind the Battle over Fen-Phen*, 1st ed. (New York: St. Martin's Press, 2002).

104. Center for Consumer Freedom, *An Epidemic of Obesity Myths* (Washington, DC: Center for Consumer Freedom, 2005).

105. Pat Lyons, "Prescription for Harm," in *The Fat Studies Reader*, ed. Esther Rothblum and Sondra Solovay (New York: New York University Press, 2009), 75–87.

106. Lucy Aphramor, "Validity of Claims Made in Weight Management Research: A Narrative Review of Dietetic Articles," *Nutrition Journal* 9 (July 20, 2010): 30.

107. Aphramor, "The Impact of a Weight-Centred Treatment Approach on Women's Health and Health-Seeking Behaviours."

108. Dawn Clifford et al., "Impact of Non-Diet Approaches on Attitudes, Behaviors, and Health Outcomes: A Systematic Review," *Journal of Nutrition Education and Behavior* 47, no. 2 (April 2015): 143–155.e1.

109. Jonas Salomonsen, "Weight Loss Does Not Prolong the Lives of Diabetes Patients," ScienceNordic, February 11, 2016, http://sciencenordic.com/weight -loss-does-not-prolong-lives-diabetes-patients.

110. Mann et al., "Medicare's Search for Effective Obesity Treatments," 230.

111. LeTourneau, "What the $60 Billion Weight Loss Industry Doesn't Want You to Know."

Chapter 3: Finding Peace

1. Linda Bacon, *Health at Every Size: The Surprising Truth about Your Weight* (Dallas: BenBella Books, 2008).

2. Jonathan Mond et al., "Quality of Life Impairment Associated with Body Dissatisfaction in a General Population Sample of Women," *BMC Public Health* 13, no. 1 (October 3, 2013): 920.

3. L. Hallberg et al., "Iron Absorption from Southeast Asian Diets. II. Role of Various Factors That Might Explain Low Absorption," *American Journal of Clinical Nutrition* 30, no. 4 (April 1977): 539–548.

4. Susan Greenhalgh, *Fat-Talk Nation: The Human Costs of America's War on Fat* (Ithaca, NY: Cornell University Press, 2015).

5. O. G. Edholm et al., "The Energy Expenditure and Food Intake of Individual Men," *British Journal of Nutrition* 9, no. 3 (1955): 286–300.

6. E. Sims, "Studies in Human Hyperphagia," in *Treatment and Management of Obesity*, ed. George A. Bray and John E. Bethune (Hagerstown, MD: Medical Dept., Harper & Row, 1974).

7. Kathy Kater, *Healthy Bodies; Teaching Kids What They Need to Know: A Comprehensive Curriculum to Address Body Image, Eating, Fitness and Weight Concerns in Today's Challenging Environment* (North St. Paul, MN: BodyImageHealth, 2012), 111–112.

8. Jon Kabat-Zinn, *Wherever You Go, There You Are: Mindfulness Meditation in Everyday Life* (New York: Hachette Books, 1994), 4.

9. Tracy L. Tylka, "Development and Psychometric Evaluation of a Measure of Intuitive Eating," *Journal of Counseling Psychology* 53, no. 2 (April 2006): 226–240.

Chapter 4: Eating 2.0: Upgrading Your Relationship with Food

1. A. Keys et al., *The Biology of Human Starvation*, 2 vols. (Oxford, England: University of Minnesota Press, 1950).

2. Brene Brown, *Women & Shame: Reaching Out, Speaking Truths and Building Connection* (Austin, TX: 3C Press, 2004), 15, 114.

3. Richard Wrangham, *Catching Fire: How Cooking Made Us Human* (New York: Basic Books, 2010).

4. Frances O'Roark Dowell, *The Second Life of Abigail Walker* (New York: Scholastic, 2012), 81.

5. Susan Greenhalgh, *Fat-Talk Nation: The Human Costs of America's War on Fat* (Ithaca, NY: Cornell University Press, 2015).

6. Anthony Warner, *The Angry Chef's Guide to Spotting Bullsh*t in the World of Food: Bad Science and the Truth about Healthy Eating*, 1st ed. (New York: The Experiment, LLC, 2018), 151.

Chapter 5: Healing the Self-Hate Injuries, Reclaiming Body Joy

1. Hanne Blank, *The Unapologetic Fat Girl's Guide to Exercise and Other Incendiary Acts* (New York: Ten Speed Press, 2012), 6.

2. Tracy L. Tylka et al., "The Weight-Inclusive versus Weight-Normative Approach to Health: Evaluating the Evidence for Prioritizing Well-Being over Weight Loss," *Journal of Obesity* (2014): 1–18.

3. Ragen Chastain, *Fat: The Owner's Manual* (Austin, TX: Sized for Success Multimedia, LLC, 2012).

4. C. E. Murphy, *Urban Shaman*, Original edition (New York: Luna, 2009), 129.

5. Paul Linden, personal communication, 2011.

6. Melanie Rawn, *Playing to the Gods*, Glass Thorns series, book 5 (New York: Tor, 2017), 347.

7. Blank, *The Unapologetic Fat Girl's Guide to Exercise and Other Incendiary Acts*.

8. Jeanette Lynn DePatie, *The Fat Chick Works Out!* (Los Angeles: Real Big Publishing, 2011).

Chapter 6: Dealing with the World: Weight Stigma, Part 1

1. Noortje van Amsterdam, "Big Fat Inequalities, Thin Privilege: An Intersectional Perspective on 'Body Size,'" *European Journal of Women's Studies* 20, no. 2 (2013): 155–169.

2. Gordon Allport, Kenneth Clark, and Thomas Pettigrew, *The Nature of Prejudice: 25th Anniversary Edition* (New York: Addison-Wesley, 1979).

3. Angela Meadows and Sigrún Daníelsdóttir, "What's in a Word? On Weight Stigma and Terminology," *Frontiers in Psychology* 7 (October 5, 2016): 1527.

4. Ragen Chastain, *Fat: The Owner's Manual* (Austin, TX: Sized for Success Multimedia, LLC, 2012).

5. Peggy Elam, personal communication, 2018.

6. Renee Engeln, *Beauty Sick: How the Cultural Obsession with Appearance Hurts Girls and Women* (New York: HarperCollins, 2017).

7. Dianne Neumark-Sztainer et al., "Does Body Satisfaction Matter? Five-Year Longitudinal Associations between Body Satisfaction and Health Behaviors in Adolescent Females and Males," *Journal of Adolescent Health: Official Publication of the Society for Adolescent Medicine* 39, no. 2 (August 2006): 244–251.

8. Dianne Neumark-Sztainer et al., "Obesity, Disordered Eating, and Eating Disorders in a Longitudinal Study of Adolescents: How Do Dieters Fare 5 Years Later?," *Journal of the American Dietetic Association* 106, no. 4 (April 2006): 559–568.

9. Lenny R. Vartanian and Jacqueline G. Shaprow, "Effects of Weight Stigma on Exercise Motivation and Behavior: A Preliminary Investigation among College-Aged Females," *Journal of Health Psychology* 13, no. 1 (January 2008): 131–138.

10. Brene Brown, *Women & Shame: Reaching Out, Speaking Truths and Building Connection* (Austin, TX: 3C Press, 2004), 15.

11. Engeln, *Beauty Sick.*

12. Sarah Addison Allen, *Lost Lake: A Novel* (New York: St. Martin's Press, 2014), 136.

13. Harriet Brown, *Body of Truth: How Science, History, and Culture Drive Our Obsession with Weight—And What We Can Do about It* (Boston, MA: Da Capo Lifelong Books, 2015).

14. Engeln, *Beauty Sick.*

15. Renee Engeln-Maddox, Rachel H. Salk, and Steven A. Miller, "Assessing Women's Negative Commentary on Their Own Bodies: A Psychometric Investigation of the Negative Body Talk Scale," *Psychology of Women Quarterly* 36, no. 2 (June 1, 2012): 162–178.

16. Renee Engeln and Rachel H Salk, "The Demographics of Fat Talk in Adult Women: Age, Body Size, and Ethnicity," *Journal of Health Psychology* 21, no. 8 (August 1, 2016): 1655–1664.

17. Anthony Warner, *The Angry Chef's Guide to Spotting Bullsh*t in the World of Food: Bad Science and the Truth about Healthy Eating*, 1st ed. (New York: The Experiment, LLC, 2018), 215.

Chapter 7: Social Justice: Weight Stigma, Part 2

1. A. Janet Tomiyama et al., "How and Why Weight Stigma Drives the Obesity 'Epidemic' and Harms Health," *BMC Medicine* 16 (August 15, 2018), 1.

2. Angela Meadows, *Fear and Self-Loathing: Internalised Weight Stigma and Maladaptive Coping in Higher-Weight Individuals.* Dissertation (University of Birmingham, 2017).

3. Ibid.

4. John F. Dovidio et al., "Physical Health Disparities and Stigma: Race, Sexual Orientation, and Body Weight," in *The Oxford Handbook of Stigma, Discrimination, and Health*, ed. Brenda Major, John F. Dovidio, and Bruce G. Link (New York: Oxford University Press, 2018), 29–52.

5. Brenda Major and Toni Schmader, "Stigma, Social Identity Threat, and Health," in *The Oxford Handbook of Stigma, Discrimination, and Health*, ed. Brenda Major, John F. Dovidio, and Bruce G. Link (New York: Oxford University Press, 2018), 85–104.

6. Jeffrey M. Hunger et al., "The Psychological and Physiological Effects of Interacting with an Anti-Fat Peer," *Body Image* 27 (December 2018): 148–155.

7. Major and Schmader, "Stigma, Social Identity Threat, and Health."

8. Jolanda Jetten, "When Discrimination Is Considered Legitimate and the Path to Illegitimacy" (4th International Weight Stigma Conference, Vancouver, Canada, 2016).

9. Jolanda Jetten et al., "Social Identity, Stigma, and Health," in *The Oxford Handbook of Stigma, Discrimination, and Health*, ed. Brenda Major, John F. Dovidio, and Bruce G. Link (New York: Oxford University Press, 2018), 301–316.

10. Dovidio et al., "Physical Health Disparities and Stigma."

11. "Project Implicit," https://implicit.harvard.edu/implicit.

12. Tessa E. S. Charlesworth and Mahzarin R. Banaji, "Patterns of Implicit and Explicit Attitudes: I. Long-Term Change and Stability from 2007 to 2016," *Psychological Science* 30, no. 2 (January 3, 2019): 174–192.

13. Stella Medvedyuk, Ahmednur Ali, and Dennis Raphael, "Ideology, Obesity and the Social Determinants of Health: A Critical Analysis of the Obesity and Health Relationship," *Critical Public Health* 28, no. 5 (October 20, 2018): 573–585.

14. Michael Marmot, *The Health Gap* (New York: Bloomsbury Press, 2015).

15. Rebecca M. Puhl and Chelsea A. Heuer, "The Stigma of Obesity: A Review and Update," *Obesity* 17, no. 5 (May 1, 2009): 941–964.

16. Gordon Allport, Kenneth Clark, and Thomas Pettigrew, *The Nature of Prejudice: 25th Anniversary Edition* (New York: Addison-Wesley, 1979).

17. Lindy West, *Shrill: Notes from a Loud Woman* (New York: Hachette Books, 2017), 72.

18. Brenda Major et al., "Stigma and Its Implications for Health: Introduction and Overview," in *The Oxford Handbook of Stigma, Discrimination, and Health*, ed. Brenda Major, John F. Dovidio, and Bruce G. Link (New York: Oxford University Press, 2018), 3–28.

19. Jetten et al., "Social Identity, Stigma, and Health."

20. Ibid.

21. Allen W. Barton and Gene H. Brody, "Parenting as a Buffer That Deters Discrimination and Race-Related Stressors from 'Getting under the Skin': Theories, Findings, and Future Directions," in *The Oxford Handbook of Stigma, Discrimination, and Health*, ed. Brenda Major, John F. Dovidio, and Bruce G. Link (New York: Oxford University Press, 2018), 335–354.

22. West, *Shrill*, 113.

23. Paula M. Brochu, "Weight Stigma Is a Modifiable Risk Factor," *Journal of Adolescent Health* 63, no. 3 (September 1, 2018): 267–268.

24. Brenda Major, Wendy Berry Mendes, and John F. Dovidio, "Intergroup Relations and Health Disparities: A Social Psychological Perspective," *Health Psychology: Official Journal of the Division of Health Psychology, American Psychological Association* 32, no. 5 (May 2013): 514–524.

25. Lenny R. Vartanian and Joshua M. Smyth, "Primum Non Nocere: Obesity Stigma and Public Health," *Journal of Bioethical Inquiry* 10, no. 1 (March 2013): 49–57.

26. A. Janet Tomiyama et al., "Associations of Weight Stigma with Cortisol and Oxidative Stress Independent of Adiposity," *Health Psychology: Official*

Journal of the Division of Health Psychology, American Psychological Association 33, no. 8 (August 2014): 862–867.

27. Tomiyama et al., "How and Why Weight Stigma Drives the Obesity 'Epidemic' and Harms Health."

28. Alicia Mundy, *Dispensing with the Truth: The Victims, the Drug Companies, and the Dramatic Story behind the Battle over Fen-Phen*, 1st ed. (New York: St. Martin's Press, 2002).

29. Brenda Major, A. Janet Tomiyama, and Jeffrey M. Hunger, "The Negative and Bidirectional Effects of Weight Stigma on Health," in *The Oxford Handbook of Stigma, Discrimination, and Health*, ed. Brenda Major, John F. Dovidio, and Bruce G. Link (New York: Oxford University Press, 2018), 499–520.

30. Puhl and Heuer, "The Stigma of Obesity."

31. N. K. Amy et al., "Barriers to Routine Gynecological Cancer Screening for White and African-American Obese Women," *International Journal of Obesity* 30, no. 1 (2006): 147–155.

32. Jennifer A. Lee and Cat J. Pausé, "Stigma in Practice: Barriers to Health for Fat Women," *Frontiers in Psychology* 7 (December 30, 2016): 1–15.

33. Janell L. Mensinger, Tracy L. Tylka, and Margaret E. Calamari, "Mechanisms Underlying Weight Status and Healthcare Avoidance in Women: A Study of Weight Stigma, Body-Related Shame and Guilt, and Healthcare Stress," *Body Image* 25 (June 2018): 139–147.

34. Puhl and Heuer, "The Stigma of Obesity."

35. "Ellen Maud Bennett," Legacy.com, July 15, 2018, https://www.legacy.com/obituaries/timescolonist/obituary.aspx?n=ellen-maud-bennett&pid=189588876.

36. Rebecca M. Puhl et al., "Weight Bias among Professionals Treating Eating Disorders: Attitudes about Treatment and Perceived Patient Outcomes," *International Journal of Eating Disorders* 47, no. 1 (January 2014): 65–75.

37. Ingemar Swenne, Thomas Parling, and Helena Salonen Ros, "Family-Based Intervention in Adolescent Restrictive Eating Disorders: Early Treatment Response and Low Weight Suppression Is Associated with Favourable One-Year Outcome," *BMC Psychiatry* 17, no. 333 (2017): 1–10.

38. American Psychiatric Association, *Diagnostic and Statistical Manual of Mental Disorders*, 5th ed. (Washington, DC: American Psychiatric Association, 2013).

39. Erin Harrop, "All Bodies Affected, Not All Bodies Accepted: Inequality of Eating Disorder Treatment for Higher Weight Populations and Solutions towards Accessibility" (Uniting against Oppression, Portland, Oregon, 2018).

40. Erin N. Harrop, "Typical-Atypical Interactions: One Patient's Experience of Weight Bias in an Inpatient Eating Disorder Treatment Setting," *Women & Therapy* 41, no. 1–2 (December 31, 2018): 1–14.

41. Sonya Renee Taylor, *The Body Is Not an Apology: The Power of Radical Self-Love* (Oakland, CA: Berrett-Koehler, 2018), 50.

42. Ibid.

43. Amy L. Fairchild and Ron Bayer, "Public Health with a Punch: Fear, Stigma, and Hard-Hitting Media Campaigns," in *The Oxford Handbook of Stigma,*

Discrimination, and Health, ed. Brenda Major, John F. Dovidio, and Bruce G. Link (New York: Oxford University Press, 2018), 429–438.

44. Rasmus Køster-Rasmussen et al., "Intentional Weight Loss and Longevity in Overweight Patients with Type 2 Diabetes: A Population-Based Cohort Study," *PLOS ONE* 11, no. 1 (January 25, 2016): e0146889.

45. J. Salomonsen, "Weight Loss Does Not Prolong the Lives of Diabetes Patients," *ScienceNordic* (February 11, 2016), http://sciencenordic.com/weight -loss-does-not-prolong-lives-diabetes-patients.

46. Dawn Clifford et al., "Impact of Non-Diet Approaches on Attitudes, Behaviors, and Health Outcomes: A Systematic Review," *Journal of Nutrition Education and Behavior* 47, no. 2 (April 2015): 143–155.

47. Rachel M. Calogero, Tracy Tylka, and Janell Mensinger, "Scientific Weightism: A View of Mainstream Weight Stigma Research through a Feminist Lens," in *Feminist Perspectives on Building a Better Psychological Science of Gender*, ed. T.-A. Roberts, N. Curtin, L. E. Duncan, and L. M. Cortina (Cham, Switzerland: Springer International Publishing, 2016), 9–28.

48. A. Charrow and D. Yerramilli, "Obesity as Disease: Metaphysical and Ethical Considerations," *Ethics, Medicine and Public Health* 7 (October 1, 2018): 74–81.

49. Lee Stoner and Jon Cornwall, "Did the American Medical Association Make the Correct Decision Classifying Obesity as a Disease?," *Australasian Medical Journal* 7, no. 11 (November 30, 2014): 462–464.

50. Naomi Wolf, *The Beauty Myth: How Images of Beauty Are Used against Women* (New York: Harper Collins, 1991), 187.

51. Tomiyama et al., "How and Why Weight Stigma Drives the Obesity 'Epidemic' and Harms Health."

52. Lily O'Hara and Jane Taylor, "Health at Every Size: A Weight-Neutral Approach for Empowerment, Resilience and Peace," *International Journal of Social Work and Human Services Practice* 2, no. 6 (December 2014): 272–282.

53. Andrea Bombak, "Obesity, Health at Every Size, and Public Health Policy," *American Journal of Public Health* 104, no. 2 (February 2014): e60–e67.

54. Fairchild and Bayer, "Public Health with a Punch."

55. E. Blacksher, "Public Health and Social Justice: An Argument against Stigma as a Tool of Health Promotion and Disease Prevention," in *The Oxford Handbook of Stigma, Discrimination, and Health*, ed. Brenda Major, John F. Dovidio, and Bruce G. Link (New York: Oxford University Press, 2018), 439–456.

56. Vartanian and Smyth, "Primum Non Nocere."

57. Institute for Clinical Systems Improvement, "Going beyond Clinical Walls: Solving Complex Problems," Robert Wood Johnson Foundation, October 2014, 2, http://www.nrhi.org/uploads/going-beyond-clinical-walls-solving-complex -problems.pdf.

58. H. Hartline-Grafton, "Food Insecurity and Obesity: Understanding the Connections," 2011, https://www.nbcdi.org/food-insecurity-and-obesity -understanding-connections.

59. April Herndon, *Fat Blame: How the War on Obesity Victimizes Women and Children* (Lawrence: University Press of Kansas, 2014).

60. Natalie Boero, "Fat Kids, Working Moms, and the 'Epidemic of Obesity': Race, Class and Mother Blame," in *The Fat Studies Reader*, ed. Esther Rothblum and Sondra Solovay (New York: NYU Press, 2009), 113.

61. Puhl and Heuer, "The Stigma of Obesity."

62. Paul Ernsberger, "Does Social Class Explain the Connection between Weight and Health?," in *The Fat Studies Reader*, ed. Esther Rothblum and Sondra Solovay (NYU Press, 2009), 25–36.

63. Major, Tomiyama, and Hunger, "The Negative and Bidirectional Effects of Weight Stigma on Health."

64. Virgie Tovar, *You Have the Right to Remain Fat* (New York: The Feminist Press at CUNY, 2018), 37.

65. Ragen Chastain, *Fat: The Owner's Manual* (Austin, TX: Sized for Success Multimedia, LLC, 2012).

66. Tracy L. Tylka et al., "The Weight-Inclusive versus Weight-Normative Approach to Health: Evaluating the Evidence for Prioritizing Well-Being over Weight Loss," research article, *Journal of Obesity* 2014 (2014): 1–18.

67. Taylor, *The Body Is Not an Apology*, 21.

68. Lucy Aphramor, "Preventing Fat Stigma and Repairing Harm: A Practical, Pragmatic, Radical Response for Advancing Weight Justice through Public Health Policy and Everyday Conversation." (6th Annual Weight Stigma Conference, Leeds, 2018).

69. Lucy Aphramor, "Glossary: Healthism," accessed November 3, 2018, https://lucyaphramor.com/dietitian/glossary.

70. John Pavlovitz, *Building a Bigger Table*. Community presentation (UCC Church, Jefferson City, MO, 2018).

Chapter 8: Going to the Doctor (and Other Adventures in Medical Care)

1. Linda Bacon, *Health at Every Size: The Surprising Truth about Your Weight* (Dallas: BenBella Books, 2008).

Chapter 9: But What about the Children?

1. Jon Robison, "Beware the 'Cockroach Effect'—Faulty Data That Will Not Die!," LinkedIn, May 9, 2016, https://www.linkedin.com/pulse/beware-cockroach-effect-faulty-data-die-jon-robison.

2. W. Wayt Gibbs, "Obesity: An Overblown Epidemic?," *Scientific American* 292, no. 6 (2005): 8.

3. Jon Robison, Carmen Cool, and E Jackson, "Helping without Harming: Kids, Eating, Weight & Health," *Absolute Advantage* 7, no. 1 (2007): 2–15.

4. Jaana Juvonen et al., "Emotional Implications of Weight Stigma across Middle School: The Role of Weight-Based Peer Discrimination," *Journal of Clinical Child and Adolescent Psychology* 46, no. 1 (February 2017): 150–158.

5. Brenda Major et al., "Stigma and Its Implications for Health: Introduction and Overview," in *The Oxford Handbook of Stigma, Discrimination, and Health*, ed.

Brenda Major, John F. Dovidio, and Bruce G. Link (New York: Oxford University Press, 2018), 3–28.

6. Allen W. Barton and Gene H. Brody, "Parenting as a Buffer That Deters Discrimination and Race-Related Stressors from 'Getting under the Skin': Theories, Findings, and Future Directions," in *The Oxford Handbook of Stigma, Discrimination, and Health*, ed. Brenda Major, John F. Dovidio, and Bruce G. Link (New York: Oxford University Press, 2018), 335–354.

7. Frédérique R. E. Smink, Daphne van Hoeken, and Hans W. Hoek, "Epidemiology of Eating Disorders: Incidence, Prevalence and Mortality Rates," *Current Psychiatry Reports* 14, no. 4 (August 2012): 406–414.

8. "Eating Disorder Statistics," Mirasol Recovery Centers, accessed December 16, 2018, https://www.mirasol.net/learning-center/eating-disorder-statistics.php.

9. Adrienne Santos-Longhurst, "Type 2 Diabetes Statistics and Facts," Healthline, September 8, 2014, https://www.healthline.com/health/type-2-diabetes/statistics.

10. Clare Harris and Brian Barraclough, "Excess Mortality of Mental Disorder," *British Journal of Psychiatry* 173, no. 1 (July 1998): 11–53.

11. Jeffrey M. Hunger and A. Janet Tomiyama, "Weight Labeling and Obesity: A Longitudinal Study of Girls Aged 10 to 19 Years," *JAMA Pediatrics* 168, no. 6 (June 2014): 579–580.

12. Dianne Neumark-Sztainer et al., "Does Body Satisfaction Matter? Five-Year Longitudinal Associations between Body Satisfaction and Health Behaviors in Adolescent Females and Males," *Journal of Adolescent Health: Official Publication of the Society for Adolescent Medicine* 39, no. 2 (August 2006): 244–251.

13. K. K. Davison and L. L. Birch, "Weight Status, Parent Reaction, and Self-Concept in Five-Year-Old Girls," *Pediatrics* 107, no. 1 (January 2001): 46–53.

14. E. Jackson, "Changing the Conversation: From 'Getting Kids Thin' to Promoting Nurturing Eating for All Children," *Absolute Advantage* 7, no. 1 (2007): 24–28.

15. Brian Wansink, Lara A. Latimer, and Lizzy Pope, "'Don't Eat So Much': How Parent Comments Relate to Female Weight Satisfaction," *Eating and Weight Disorders* 22, no. 3 (September 2017): 475–481.

16. Eric Stice and Mark J. Van Ryzin, "A Prospective Test of the Temporal Sequencing of Risk Factor Emergence in the Dual Pathway Model of Eating Disorders," *Journal of Abnormal Psychology* 128, no. 2 (December 20, 2018): 119–128.

17. Yafu Zhao and William Encinosa, "An Update on Hospitalizations for Eating Disorders, 1999 to 2009: Statistical Brief #120," in *Healthcare Cost and Utilization Project (HCUP) Statistical Briefs* (Rockville, MD: Agency for Healthcare Research and Quality, 2006).

18. Dianne Neumark-Sztainer et al., "Obesity, Disordered Eating, and Eating Disorders in a Longitudinal Study of Adolescents: How Do Dieters Fare 5 Years Later?," *Journal of the American Dietetic Association* 106, no. 4 (April 2006): 559–568.

19. Susan Greenhalgh, "Weighty Subjects: The Biopolitics of the U.S. War on Fat," *American Ethnologist* 39, no. 3 (August 1, 2012): 471–487, 483.

20. Ibid., 484.

21. Neville H. Golden, Marcie Schneider, and Christine Wood, "Preventing Obesity and Eating Disorders in Adolescents," *Pediatrics* 138, no. 3 (September 1, 2016): e20161649.

22. Neumark-Sztainer et al., "Obesity, Disordered Eating, and Eating Disorders in a Longitudinal Study of Adolescents."

23. Golden, Schneider, and Wood, "Preventing Obesity and Eating Disorders in Adolescents."

24. Robison, Cool, and Jackson, "Helping without Harming."

25. Susan Yeh, "Laws and Social Norms: Unintended Consequences of Obesity Laws," *University of Cincinnati Law Review* 81 (2013): 52.

26. Joanne Ikeda, Patricia Crawford, and Gail Woodward-Lopez, "BMI Screening in Schools: Helpful or Harmful," *Health Education Research Theory & Practice* 21 (2006): 761–769.

27. Dianne Neumark-Sztainer et al., "Accurate Parental Classification of Overweight Adolescents' Weight Status: Does It Matter?," *Pediatrics* 121, no. 6 (June 2008): e1495–e1502.

28. Helene Keery et al., "The Impact of Appearance-Related Teasing by Family Members," *Journal of Adolescent Health: Official Publication of the Society for Adolescent Medicine* 37, no. 2 (August 2005): 120–127.

29. Sigrún Daníelsdóttir, Deb Burgard, and Wendy Oliver-Pyatt, "AED Guidelines for Childhood Obesity Prevention Programs," Academy for Eating Disorders, n.d., http://www.cope-ecf.org/aed-guidelines.

30. Rebecca M. Puhl et al., "Weight Stigmatization and Bias Reduction: Perspectives of Overweight and Obese Adults," *Health Education Research* 23, no. 2 (April 2008): 347–358.

Chapter 11: Final Thoughts

1. Native deodorant packaging insert, *#GoNative*, n.d.

Bibliography

Allen, Sarah Addison. *Lost Lake: A Novel*. New York: St. Martin's Press, 2014.

Allport, Gordon, Kenneth Clark, and Thomas Pettigrew. *The Nature of Prejudice: 25th Anniversary Edition*. New York: Addison-Wesley, 1979.

American Psychiatric Association. *Diagnostic and Statistical Manual of Mental Disorders*. 3rd rev. ed. Washington, DC: American Psychiatric Association, 1987.

American Psychiatric Association. *Diagnostic and Statistical Manual of Mental Disorders*. 5th ed. Washington, DC: American Psychiatric Association, 2013.

Amsterdam, Noortje van. "Big Fat Inequalities, Thin Privilege: An Intersectional Perspective on 'Body Size.'" *European Journal of Women's Studies* 20, no. 2 (2013): 155–169.

Amy, N. K., A. Aalborg, P. Lyons, and L. Keranen. "Barriers to Routine Gynecological Cancer Screening for White and African-American Obese Women." *International Journal of Obesity* 30, no. 1 (2006): 147–155.

Aphramor, Lucy. "Glossary: Healthism." Accessed November 3, 2018. https://lucyaphramor.com/dietitian/glossary/.

Aphramor, Lucy. "The Impact of a Weight-Centred Treatment Approach on Women's Health and Health-Seeking Behaviours." *Journal of Critical Dietetics* 1, no. 2 (2012): 3–12.

Aphramor, Lucy. "Preventing Fat Stigma and Repairing Harm: A Practical, Pragmatic, Radical Response for Advancing Weight Justice through Public Health Policy and Everyday Conversation." Conference. Leeds, 2018.

Aphramor, Lucy. "Validity of Claims Made in Weight Management Research: A Narrative Review of Dietetic Articles." *Nutrition Journal* 9 (July 20, 2010): 30.

Bacon, L., J. S. Stern, N. L. Keim, and M. D. Van Loan. "Low Bone Mass in Premenopausal Chronic Dieting Obese Women." *European Journal of Clinical Nutrition* 58, no. 6 (June 2004): 966–971.

Bacon, Linda. *Health at Every Size: The Surprising Truth about Your Weight*. Dallas: BenBella Books, 2008.

Bacon, Linda, and Lucy Aphramor. *Body Respect: What Conventional Health Books Get Wrong, Leave Out, and Just Plain Fail to Understand about Weight*. 1st ed. Dallas: BenBella Books, 2014.

Bacon, Linda, and Lucy Aphramor. "Weight Science: Evaluating the Evidence for a Paradigm Shift." *Nutrition Journal* 10, no. 9 (2011): 1–13.

Bacon, Linda, Judith S. Stern, Marta D. Van Loan, and Nancy L. Keim. "Size Acceptance and Intuitive Eating Improve Health for Obese, Female Chronic Dieters." *Journal of the American Dietetic Association* 105, no. 6 (June 2005): 929–936.

Bangalore, Sripal, Rana Fayyad, Rachel Laskey, David A. DeMicco, Franz H. Messerli, and David D. Waters. "Body-Weight Fluctuations and Outcomes in Coronary Disease." *New England Journal of Medicine* 376, no. 14 (April 6, 2017): 1332–1340.

Barker, Robert. *The Social Work Dictionary.* 6th ed. Washington, DC: NASW Press, 2014.

Barton, Allen W., and Gene H. Brody. "Parenting as a Buffer That Deters Discrimination and Race-Related Stressors from 'Getting Under the Skin': Theories, Findings, and Future Directions." In *The Oxford Handbook of Stigma, Discrimination, and Health,* edited by Brenda Major, John F. Dovidio, and Bruce G. Link, 335–354. New York: Oxford University Press, 2018.

Becofsky, K., X. Sui, D. Lee, S. Wilcox, J. Zhang, and S. Blair. "A Prospective Study of Fitness, Fatness, and Depressive Symptoms." *American Journal of Epidemiology* 181, no. 5 (2015): 311–320.

Bennett, William, and Joel Gurin. *The Dieter's Dilemma Eating Less and Weighing More.* New York: Basic Books, 1982.

Benton, David. "The Plausibility of Sugar Addiction and Its Role in Obesity and Eating Disorders." *Clinical Nutrition (Edinburgh, Scotland)* 29, no. 3 (June 2010): 288–303.

Berg, Frances M. *Children and Teens Afraid to Eat: Helping Youth in Today's Weight-Obsessed World.* 3rd ed. Hettinger, ND: Healthy Weight Publishing Network, 2000.

Berg, Frances M. *Women Afraid to Eat: Breaking Free in Today's Weight-Obsessed World.* 1st ed. Hettinger, ND: Healthy Weight Publishing Network, 1999.

Blacksher, E. "Public Health and Social Justice: An Argument against Stigma as a Tool of Health Promotion and Disease Prevention." In *The Oxford Handbook of Stigma, Discrimination, and Health,* edited by Brenda Major, John F. Dovidio, and Bruce G. Link, 439–456. New York: Oxford University Press, 2018.

Blake, Christine E., James R. Hébert, Duck-Chul Lee, Swann A. Adams, Susan E. Steck, Xuemei Sui, Jennifer L. Kuk, Meghan Baruth, and Steven N. Blair. "Adults with Greater Weight Satisfaction Report More Positive Health Behaviors and Have Better Health Status Regardless of BMI." *Journal of Obesity* 2013 (2013): 291371.

Blank, Hanne. *The Unapologetic Fat Girl's Guide to Exercise and Other Incendiary Acts.* Berkeley, CA: Ten Speed Press, 2012.

Boero, Natalie. "Fat Kids, Working Moms, and the 'Epidemic of Obesity': Race, Class and Mother Blame." In *The Fat Studies Reader,* edited by Esther Rothblum and Sondra Solovay, 113–119. New York: NYU Press, 2009.

Boero, Natalie. *Killer Fat: Media, Medicine, and Morals in the American "Obesity Epidemic."* New Brunswick, NJ: Rutgers University Press, 2013.

Bombak, Andrea. "Obesity, Health at Every Size, and Public Health Policy." *American Journal of Public Health* 104, no. 2 (February 2014): e60–e67.

Bordo, Susan. *Unbearable Weight: Feminism, Western Culture, and the Body, Tenth Anniversary Edition.* Berkeley: University of California Press, 2004.

Brochu, Paula M. "Weight Stigma Is a Modifiable Risk Factor." *Journal of Adolescent Health* 63, no. 3 (September 1, 2018): 267–268.

Brown, Brene. *Women & Shame: Reaching Out, Speaking Truths and Building Connection.* Austin, TX: 3C Press, 2004.

Brown, Harriet. *Body of Truth: How Science, History, and Culture Drive Our Obsession with Weight—And What We Can Do about It.* Boston: Da Capo Lifelong Books, 2015.

Brumberg, Joan Jacobs. *The Body Project: An Intimate History of American Girls.* 1st ed. New York: Vintage, 1998.

Calogero, Rachel M., Tracy Tylka, and Janell Mensinger. "Scientific Weightism: A View of Mainstream Weight Stigma Research through a Feminist Lens." In *Feminist Perspectives on Building a Better Psychological Science of Gender*, edited by Tomi-Ann Roberts, Nicola Curtin, Lauren E. Duncan, and Lilia M. Cortina, 9–28. Switzerland: Springer, 2016.

Campos, Paul. *The Obesity Myth: Why America's Obsessions with Weight Is Hazardous to Your Health.* New York: Gotham, 2005.

Center for Consumer Freedom. *An Epidemic of Obesity Myths.* Washington, DC: The Center for Consumer Freedom, 2005.

Charlesworth, Tessa E. S., and Mahzarin R. Banaji. "Patterns of Implicit and Explicit Attitudes: I. Long-Term Change and Stability from 2007 to 2016." *Psychological Science* (January 3, 2019): 174–192.

Charrow, A., and D. Yerramilli. "Obesity as Disease: Metaphysical and Ethical Considerations." *Ethics, Medicine and Public Health* 7 (October 1, 2018): 74–81.

Chastain, Ragen. *Fat: The Owner's Manual.* Austin, TX: Sized for Success Multimedia, LLC, 2012.

Chastain, Ragen, ed. *The Politics of Size: Perspectives from the Fat Acceptance Movement.* 2 vols. Santa Barbara, CA: Praeger, 2014.

Clifford, Dawn, Amy Ozier, Joanna Bundros, Jeffrey Moore, Anna Kreiser, and Michelle Neyman Morris. "Impact of Non-Diet Approaches on Attitudes, Behaviors, and Health Outcomes: A Systematic Review." *Journal of Nutrition Education and Behavior* 47, no. 2 (April 2015): 143–155.

Cooke, Kaz. *Real Gorgeous: The Truth about Body and Beauty.* St. Leonards, N.S.W.: Allen & Unwin, 1997.

Corwin, Rebecca L. W., and John E. Hayes. "Are Sugars Addictive? Perspectives for Practitioners." In *Fructose, High Fructose Corn Syrup, Sucrose and Health*, edited by James M. Rippe, 199–215. Nutrition and Health. New York: Springer New York, 2014.

Daníelsdóttir, Sigrún, Deb Burgard, and Wendy Oliver-Pyatt. "AED Guidelines for Childhood Obesity Prevention Programs." *Academy for Eating Disorders*, n.d. http://www.cope-ecf.org/aed-guidelines.

Davison, K. K., and L. L. Birch. "Weight Status, Parent Reaction, and Self-Concept in Five-Year-Old Girls." *Pediatrics* 107, no. 1 (January 2001): 46–53.

DePatie, Jeanette Lynn. *The Fat Chick Works Out!* Los Angeles: Real Big Publishing, 2011.

deShazo, Richard D., John E. Hall, and Leigh Baldwin Skipworth. "Obesity Bias, Medical Technology, and the Hormonal Hypothesis: Should We Stop Demonizing Fat People?" *American Journal of Medicine* 128, no. 5 (May 2015): 456–460.

Dollar, Emily, Margit Berman, and Anna M. Adachi-Mejia. "Do No Harm: Moving beyond Weight Loss to Emphasize Physical Activity at Every Size." *Preventing Chronic Disease* 14 (2017): E34.

Domoff, Sarah E., Nova G. Hinman, Afton M. Koball, Amy Storfer-Isser, Victoria L. Carhart, Kyoung D. Baik, and Robert A. Carels. "The Effects of Reality Television on Weight Bias: An Examination of *The Biggest Loser.*" *Obesity* (Silver Spring, MD) 20, no. 5 (May 2012): 993–998.

Dotinga, Randy. "The Average Americans' Weight Change since the 1980s Is Startling." CBS News, August 3, 2016. https://www.cbsnews.com/news /americans-weight-gain-since-1980s-startling.

Dovidio, John F., Louis A. Penner, Sarah K. Calabrese, and Rebecca L. Pearl. "Physical Health Disparities and Stigma: Race, Sexual Orientation, and Body Weight." In *The Oxford Handbook of Stigma, Discrimination, and Health*, edited by Brenda Major, John F. Dovidio, and Bruce G. Link, 29–52. New York: Oxford University Press, 2018.

Dowell, Frances O'Roark. *The Second Life of Abigail Walker.* New York: Scholastic, 2012.

Dulloo, A. G., J. Jacquet, J.-P. Montani, and Y. Schutz. "How Dieting Makes the Lean Fatter: From a Perspective of Body Composition Autoregulation through Adipostats and Proteinstats Awaiting Discovery." *Obesity Reviews: An Official Journal of the International Association for the Study of Obesity* 16, Suppl. 1 (February 2015): 25–35.

"Eating Disorder Statistics." Mirasol Recovery Centers, n.d. https://www.mirasol .net/learning-center/eating-disorder-statistics.php.

Edholm, O. G., J. G. Fletcher, E. M. Widdowson, and R. A. McCance. "The Energy Expenditure and Food Intake of Individual Men." *British Journal of Nutrition* 9, no. 3 (1955): 286–300.

Eisenberg, Marla E., Jerica M. Berge, and Dianne Neumark-Sztainer. "Dieting and Encouragement to Diet by Significant Others: Associations with Disordered Eating in Young Adults." *American Journal of Health Promotion* 27, no. 6 (August 2013): 370–377.

"Ellen Maud Bennett." Legacy.com, July 15, 2018. https://www.legacy.com/obitu aries/timescolonist/obituary.aspx?n=ellen-maud-bennett&pid=189588876.

Engeln, Renee. *Beauty Sick: How the Cultural Obsession with Appearance Hurts Girls and Women.* New York: HarperCollins, 2017.

Engeln, Renee, and Rachel H. Salk. "The Demographics of Fat Talk in Adult Women: Age, Body Size, and Ethnicity." *Journal of Health Psychology* 21, no. 8 (August 1, 2016): 1655–1664.

Engeln-Maddox, Renee, Rachel H. Salk, and Steven A. Miller. "Assessing Women's Negative Commentary on Their Own Bodies: A Psychometric Investigation of the Negative Body Talk Scale." *Psychology of Women Quarterly* 36, no. 2 (June 1, 2012): 162–178.

Ernsberger, Paul. "Does Social Class Explain the Connection between Weight and Health?" In *The Fat Studies Reader*, edited by Esther Rothblum and Sondra Solovay, 25–36. New York: NYU Press, 2009.

Fairchild, Amy L., and Ron Bayer. "Public Health with a Punch: Fear, Stigma, and Hard-Hitting Media Campaigns." In *The Oxford Handbook of Stigma, Discrimination, and Health*, edited by Brenda Major, John F. Dovidio, and Bruce G. Link, 429–438. New York: Oxford University Press, 2018.

Farrell, Amy Erdman. *Fat Shame: Stigma and the Fat Body in American Culture.* 2nd printing ed. New York: NYU Press, 2011.

Fell, James. "'It's a Miracle No One Has Died Yet': The Biggest Loser Returns, Despite Critics' Warnings." *The Guardian*, January 4, 2016. https://www.theguardian.com/tv-and-radio/2016/jan/04/the-biggest-loser-returns-despite-critics-warnings.

Fildes, Alison, Judith Charlton, Caroline Rudisill, Peter Littlejohns, A. Toby Prevost, and Martin C. Gulliford. "Probability of an Obese Person Attaining Normal Body Weight: Cohort Study Using Electronic Health Records." *American Journal of Public Health* 105, no. 9 (September 2015): e54–e59.

Flegal, Katherine M., Brian K. Kit, Heather Orpana, and Barry I. Graubard. "Association of All-Cause Mortality with Overweight and Obesity Using Standard Body Mass Index Categories: A Systematic Review and Meta-Analysis." *JAMA* 309, no. 1 (January 2, 2013): 71–82.

Fothergill, Erin, Juen Guo, Lilian Howard, Jennifer C. Kerns, Nicolas D. Knuth, Robert Brychta, Kong Y. Chen, et al. "Persistent Metabolic Adaptation 6 Years after 'The Biggest Loser' Competition." *Obesity* 24, no. 8 (2016): 1612–1619.

Fraser, Laura. *Losing It: False Hopes and Fat Profits in the Diet Industry.* New York: Plume, 1998.

Freedman, Rita. *Beauty Bound.* 1st ed. Lexington, MA: Prentice Hall & IBD, 1985.

Freedman, Rita. *Bodylove: Learning to Like Our Looks and Ourselves: A Practical Guide for Women.* Carlsbad, CA: Gurze Books, 2002.

Gaesser, Glenn A. *Big Fat Lies: The Truth about Your Weight and Your Health.* 1st trade paper ed. Carlsbad, CA: Gurze Books, 2002.

Gapinski, Katherine D., Kelly D. Brownell, and Marianne LaFrance. "Body Objectification and 'Fat Talk': Effects on Emotion, Motivation, and Cognitive Performance." *Sex Roles* 48, no. 9–10 (2003): 377–388.

Garner, David M., and Susan C. Wooley. "Confronting the Failure of Behavioral and Dietary Treatments for Obesity." *Clinical Psychology Review* 11, no. 6 (1991): 729–780.

Gibbs, W. Wayt. "Obesity: An Overblown Epidemic?" *Scientific American* 292, no. 6 (2005): 70–77.

Golden, Neville H., Marcie Schneider, and Christine Wood. "Preventing Obesity and Eating Disorders in Adolescents." *Pediatrics* 138, no. 3 (2016): e20161649.

Greenhalgh, Susan. *Fat-Talk Nation: The Human Costs of America's War on Fat.* Ithaca, NY: Cornell University Press, 2015.

Greenhalgh, Susan. "Weighty Subjects: The Biopolitics of the U.S. War on Fat." *American Ethnologist* 39, no. 3 (August 1, 2012): 471–487.

Grodstein, F., R. Levine, L. Troy, T. Spencer, G. A. Colditz, and M. J. Stampfer. "Three-Year Follow-Up of Participants in a Commercial Weight Loss Program. Can You Keep It Off?" *Archives of Internal Medicine* 156, no. 12 (June 24, 1996): 1302–1306.

Hallberg, L., E. Björn-Rasmussen, L. Rossander, and R. Suwanik. "Iron Absorption from Southeast Asian Diets. II. Role of Various Factors That Might Explain Low Absorption." *American Journal of Clinical Nutrition* 30, no. 4 (April 1977): 539–548.

Harris, Clare, and Brian Barraclough. "Excess Mortality of Mental Disorder." *British Journal of Psychiatry* 173, no. 1 (July 1998): 11–53.

Harrop, Erin. "All Bodies Affected, Not All Bodies Accepted: Inequality of Eating Disorder Treatment for Higher Weight Populations and Solutions towards Accessibility." Lecture. Portland, OR, 2018.

Harrop, Erin N. "Typical-Atypical Interactions: One Patient's Experience of Weight Bias in an Inpatient Eating Disorder Treatment Setting." *Women & Therapy* 41, no. 1–2 (December 31, 2018): 45–58.

Hartline-Grafton, H. "Food Insecurity and Obesity: Understanding the Connections," National Black Child Development Institute, 2011. https://www.nbcdi.org/food-insecurity-and-obesity-understanding-connections.

Hatzenbuehler, Mark L. "Structural Stigma and Health." In *The Oxford Handbook of Stigma, Discrimination, and Health*, edited by Brenda Major, John F. Dovidio, and Bruce G. Link, 105–124. New York: Oxford University Press, 2018.

Herndon, April. *Fat Blame: How the War on Obesity Victimizes Women and Children.* Lawrence: University Press of Kansas, 2014.

Hirschmann, Jane R., and Carol H. Munter. *Overcoming Overeating: How to Break the Diet/Binge Cycle and Live a Healthier, More Satisfying Life.* New York: OO Publishing, 2010.

Hirschmann, Jane R., and Carol H. Munter. *When Women Stop Hating Their Bodies: Freeing Yourself from Food and Weight Obsession.* 1st ed. New York: Ballantine Books, 1996.

Hunger, Jeffrey M., Alison Blodorn, Carol T. Miller, and Brenda Major. "The Psychological and Physiological Effects of Interacting with an Anti-Fat Peer." *Body Image* 27 (December 2018): 148–155.

Hunger, Jeffrey M., and A. Janet Tomiyama. "Weight Labeling and Obesity: A Longitudinal Study of Girls Aged 10 to 19 Years." *JAMA Pediatrics* 168, no. 6 (June 2014): 579–580.

Ikeda, Joanne, Patricia Crawford, and Gail Woodward-Lopez. "BMI Screening in Schools: Helpful or Harmful." *Health Education Research Theory & Practice* 21 (2006): 761–769.

Institute for Clinical Systems Improvement. "Going beyond Clinical Walls: Solving Complex Problems." Robert Wood Johnson Foundation, October 2014, 2.

Jackson, E. "Changing the Conversation: From 'Getting Kids Thin' to Promoting Nurturing Eating for All Children." *Absolute Advantage* 7, no. 1 (2007): 24–28.

Jetten, Jolanda. "When Discrimination Is Considered Legitimate and the Path to Illegitimacy." Lecture. Vancouver, Canada, 2016.

Jetten, Jolanda, S. Alexander Haslam, Tegan Cruwys, and Nyla R. Branscombe. "Social Identity, Stigma, and Health." In *The Oxford Handbook of Stigma, Discrimination, and Health*, edited by Brenda Major, John F. Dovidio, and Bruce G. Link, 301–316. New York: Oxford University Press, 2018.

Juvonen, Jaana, Leah M. Lessard, Hannah L. Schacter, and Luisana Suchilt. "Emotional Implications of Weight Stigma across Middle School: The Role of Weight-Based Peer Discrimination." *Journal of Clinical Child and Adolescent Psychology* 46, no. 1 (February 2017): 150–158.

Kabat-Zinn, Jon. *Wherever You Go, There You Are: Mindfulness Meditation in Everyday Life*. New York: Hachette Books, 1994.

Karsay, Kathrin, and Desirée Schmuck. "'Weak, Sad, and Lazy Fatties': Adolescents' Explicit and Implicit Weight Bias Following Exposure to Weight Loss Reality TV Shows." *Media Psychology* 22, no. 1 (January 2, 2019): 60–81.

Kater, Kathy. *Healthy Bodies; Teaching Kids What They Need to Know: A Comprehensive Curriculum to Address Body Image, Eating, Fitness and Weight Concerns in Today's Challenging Environment*. North St. Paul, MN: BodyImageHealth, 2012.

Kater, Kathy J. "Why 'Obesity Prevention' Is Making Us Fatter, More Poorly Nourished, and Less Fit—The Need for a New Paradigm for Weight." BodyImageHealth.org, 2010. https://www.sizediversityandhealth.org/images/uploaded/Kater%20-%20White%20Paper,%20pdf.pdf.

Kater, Kathy J., John Rohwer, and Karen Londre. "Evaluation of an Upper Elementary School Program to Prevent Body Image, Eating, and Weight Concerns." *Journal of School Health* 72, no. 5 (May 2002): 199–204.

Keery, Helene, Kerri Boutelle, Patricia van den Berg, and J. Kevin Thompson. "The Impact of Appearance-Related Teasing by Family Members." *Journal of Adolescent Health: Official Publication of the Society for Adolescent Medicine* 37, no. 2 (August 2005): 120–127.

Kelly, Amy M., Melanie Wall, Marla E. Eisenberg, Mary Story, and Dianne Neumark-Sztainer. "Adolescent Girls with High Body Satisfaction: Who Are They and What Can They Teach Us?" *Journal of Adolescent Health: Official Publication of the Society for Adolescent Medicine* 37, no. 5 (November 2005): 391–396.

Keys, A., J. Brožek, A. Henschel, O. Mickelsen, and H. L. Taylor. *The Biology of Human Starvation*. 2 vols. Oxford, England: University of Minnesota Press, 1950.

Kim, Mee Kyoung, Kyungdo Han, Yong-Moon Park, Hyuk-Sang Kwon, Gunseog Kang, Kun-Ho Yoon, and Seung-Hwan Lee. "Associations of Variability in Blood Pressure, Glucose and Cholesterol Concentrations, and Body Mass Index with Mortality and Cardiovascular Outcomes in the General Population." *Circulation* 138, no. 23 (December 4, 2018): 2627–2637.

Køster-Rasmussen, Rasmus, Mette Kildevæld Simonsen, Volkert Siersma, Jan Erik Henriksen, Berit Lilienthal Heitmann, and Niels de Fine Olivarius. "Intentional Weight Loss and Longevity in Overweight Patients with Type 2 Diabetes: A Population-Based Cohort Study." *PLOS ONE* 11, no. 1 (January 25, 2016): e0146889.

Lee, Jennifer A., and Cat J. Pausé. "Stigma in Practice: Barriers to Health for Fat Women." *Frontiers in Psychology* 7 (December 30, 2016).

Leibel, R. L., M. Rosenbaum, and J. Hirsch. "Changes in Energy Expenditure Resulting from Altered Body Weight." *New England Journal of Medicine* 332, no. 10 (March 9, 1995): 621–628.

LeTourneau, Nancy. "What the $60 Billion Weight Loss Industry Doesn't Want You to Know," *Washington Monthly*, May 2, 2016. https://washington monthly.com/2016/05/02/what-the-60-billion-weight-loss-industry -doesnt-want-you-to-know.

Levenstein, Harvey. *Revolution at the Table: The Transformation of the American Diet*. 1st ed. Berkeley: University of California Press, 2003.

Lyons, Pat. "Prescription for Harm." In *The Fat Studies Reader*, 75–87. New York: New York University Press, 2009.

Lyons, Pat, and Debby Burgard. *Great Shape: The First Exercise Guide for Large Women*. 1st ed. New York: Arbor House Pub Co, 1988.

Macpherson-Sánchez, Ann E. "Integrating Fundamental Concepts of Obesity and Eating Disorders: Implications for the Obesity Epidemic." *American Journal of Public Health* 105, no. 4 (April 2015): e71–e85.

Major, Brenda, John F. Dovidio, Bruce G. Link, and Sarah K. Calabrese. "Stigma and Its Implications for Health: Introduction and Overview." In *The Oxford Handbook of Stigma, Discrimination, and Health*, edited by Brenda Major, John F. Dovidio, and Bruce G. Link, 3–28. New York: Oxford University Press, 2018.

Major, Brenda, Wendy Berry Mendes, and John F. Dovidio. "Intergroup Relations and Health Disparities: A Social Psychological Perspective." *Health Psychology: Official Journal of the Division of Health Psychology, American Psychological Association* 32, no. 5 (May 2013): 514–524.

Major, Brenda, and Toni Schmader. "Stigma, Social Identity Threat, and Health." In *The Oxford Handbook of Stigma, Discrimination, and Health*, edited by Brenda Major, John F. Dovidio, and Bruce G. Link, 85–104. New York: Oxford University Press, 2018.

Major, Brenda, A. Janet Tomiyama, and Jeffrey M. Hunger. "The Negative and Bidirectional Effects of Weight Stigma on Health." In *The Oxford Handbook of Stigma, Discrimination, and Health*, edited by Brenda Major, John F. Dovidio, and Bruce G. Link, 499–520. New York: Oxford University Press, 2018.

Mann, Traci. *Secrets from the Eating Lab.* New York: HarperCollins, 2015.

Mann, Traci, A. Janet Tomiyama, and Andrew Ward. "Promoting Public Health in the Context of the 'Obesity Epidemic': False Starts and Promising New Directions." *Perspectives on Psychological Science: A Journal of the Association for Psychological Science* 10, no. 6 (November 2015): 706–710.

Mann, Traci, A. Janet Tomiyama, Erika Westling, Ann-Marie Lew, Barbra Samuels, and Jason Chatman. "Medicare's Search for Effective Obesity Treatments: Diets Are Not the Answer." *American Psychologist* 62, no. 3 (April 2007): 220–233.

Marmot, Michael. *The Health Gap.* New York: Bloomsbury Press, 2015.

Matheson, Eric M., Dana E. King, and Charles J. Everett. "Healthy Lifestyle Habits and Mortality in Overweight and Obese Individuals." *Journal of the American Board of Family Medicine* 25, no. 1 (February 2012): 9–15.

Matz, Judith. "Health Comes in All Sizes: The HAES Approach to Countering Weight Stigma." *Psychotherapy Networker* (November/December 2018): 17–19.

Matz, Judith, and Ellen Frankel. *Beyond a Shadow of a Diet: The Therapist's Guide to Treating Compulsive Eating Disorders.* 1st ed. New York: Routledge, 2004.

Matz, Judith, and Ellen Frankel. *The Diet Survivor's Handbook: 60 Lessons in Eating, Acceptance and Self-Care.* Naperville, IL: Sourcebooks, 2006.

Meadows, Angela. "Fear and Self-Loathing: Internalised Weight Stigma and Maladaptive Coping in Higher-Weight Individuals." Dissertation. University of Birmingham, 2017.

Meadows, Angela, and Sigrún Daníelsdóttir. "What's in a Word? On Weight Stigma and Terminology." *Frontiers in Psychology* 7 (October 5, 2016).

Meadows, Angela, Laurence J. Nolan, and Suzanne Higgs. "Self-Perceived Food Addiction: Prevalence, Predictors, and Prognosis." *Appetite* 114: 282–298.

Medvedyuk, Stella, Ahmednur Ali, and Dennis Raphael. "Ideology, Obesity and the Social Determinants of Health: A Critical Analysis of the Obesity and Health Relationship." *Critical Public Health* 28, no. 5 (October 20, 2018): 573–585.

Mensinger, Janell L., Tracy L. Tylka, and Margaret E. Calamari. "Mechanisms Underlying Weight Status and Healthcare Avoidance in Women: A Study of Weight Stigma, Body-Related Shame and Guilt, and Healthcare Stress." *Body Image* 25 (June 2018): 139–147.

Mond, Jonathan, Deborah Mitchison, Janet Latner, Phillipa Hay, Cathy Owen, and Bryan Rodgers. "Quality of Life Impairment Associated with Body Dissatisfaction in a General Population Sample of Women." *BMC Public Health* 13, no. 1 (October 3, 2013): 920.

Muennig, Peter. "The Body Politic: The Relationship between Stigma and Obesity-Associated Disease." *BMC Public Health* 8 (April 21, 2008): 128.

Muennig, Peter, Haomiao Jia, Rufina Lee, and Erica Lubetkin. "I Think Therefore I Am: Perceived Ideal Weight as a Determinant of Health." *American Journal of Public Health* 98, no. 3 (March 2008): 501–506.

Mundy, Alicia. *Dispensing with the Truth: The Victims, the Drug Companies, and the Dramatic Story behind the Battle over Fen-Phen*. 1st ed. New York: St. Martin's Press, 2002.

Murphy, C. E. *Urban Shaman*. Original ed. New York: Luna, 2009.

Native. Deodorant packaging insert. #GoNative, n.d.

Neumark-Sztainer, Dianne. "Preventing Obesity and Eating Disorders in Adolescents: What Can Health Care Providers Do?" *Journal of Adolescent Health: Official Publication of the Society for Adolescent Medicine* 44, no. 3 (March 2009): 206–213.

Neumark-Sztainer, Dianne, Susan J. Paxton, Peter J. Hannan, Jess Haines, and Mary Story. "Does Body Satisfaction Matter? Five-Year Longitudinal Associations between Body Satisfaction and Health Behaviors in Adolescent Females and Males." *Journal of Adolescent Health: Official Publication of the Society for Adolescent Medicine* 39, no. 2 (August 2006): 244–251.

Neumark-Sztainer, Dianne, Melanie Wall, Jia Guo, Mary Story, Jess Haines, and Marla Eisenberg. "Obesity, Disordered Eating, and Eating Disorders in a Longitudinal Study of Adolescents: How Do Dieters Fare 5 Years Later?" *Journal of the American Dietetic Association* 106, no. 4 (April 2006): 559–568.

Neumark-Sztainer, Dianne, Melanie Wall, Mary Story, and Patricia van den Berg. "Accurate Parental Classification of Overweight Adolescents' Weight Status: Does It Matter?" *Pediatrics* 121, no. 6 (June 2008): e1495–e1502.

Ochner, Christopher N., Adam G. Tsai, Robert F. Kushner, and Thomas A. Wadden. "Treating Obesity Seriously: When Recommendations for Lifestyle Change Confront Biological Adaptations." *Lancet Diabetes & Endocrinology* 3, no. 4 (April 1, 2015): 232–234.

O'Hara, Lily, and Jane Gregg. "The War on Obesity: A Social Determinant of Health." *Health Promotion Journal of Australia: Official Journal of Australian Association of Health Promotion Professionals* 17, no. 3 (December 2006): 260–263.

O'Hara, Lily, and Jane Taylor. "Health at Every Size: A Weight-Neutral Approach for Empowerment, Resilience and Peace." *International Journal of Social Work and Human Services Practice* 2, no. 6 (December 2014): 272–282.

Oliver, J. Eric. *Fat Politics: The Real Story behind America's Obesity Epidemic*. New York: Oxford University Press, 2006.

Oliver, J. Eric. "The Politics of Pathology: How Obesity Became an Epidemic Disease." *Perspectives in Biology and Medicine* 49, no. 4 (2006): 611–627.

Pause, Cat. "Die Another Day: The Obstacles Facing Fat People in Accessing Quality Healthcare." *Narrative Inquiry in Bioethics* 4, no. 2 (2014): 135–141.

Pavlovitz, John. *Building a Bigger Table*. Community presentation. Jefferson City, MO, 2018.

Pershing, Amy, and Chevese Turner. *Binge Eating Disorder: The Journey to Recovery and Beyond.* 1st ed. New York: Routledge, 2018.

Pratchett, Terry. *Going Postal.* London: Doubleday, 2004.

"Project Implicit." Accessed January 12, 2019. https://implicit.harvard.edu/implicit.

Puhl, R., J. L. Peterson, and J. Luedicke. "Fighting Obesity or Obese Persons? Public Perceptions of Obesity-Related Health Messages." *International Journal of Obesity* 37, no. 6 (June 2013): 774–782.

Puhl, Rebecca M., and Kelly D. Brownell. "Confronting and Coping with Weight Stigma: An Investigation of Overweight and Obese Adults." *Obesity* (Silver Spring, MD) 14, no. 10 (October 2006): 1802–1815.

Puhl, Rebecca M., and Chelsea A. Heuer. "Obesity Stigma: Important Considerations for Public Health." *American Journal of Public Health* 100, no. 6 (2010): 1019–1028.

Puhl, Rebecca M., and Chelsea A. Heuer. "The Stigma of Obesity: A Review and Update." *Obesity* 17, no. 5 (May 1, 2009): 941–964.

Puhl, Rebecca M., Janet D. Latner, Kelly M. King, and Joerg Luedicke. "Weight Bias among Professionals Treating Eating Disorders: Attitudes about Treatment and Perceived Patient Outcomes." *International Journal of Eating Disorders* 47, no. 1 (January 2014): 65–75.

Puhl, Rebecca M., Corinne A. Moss-Racusin, Marlene B. Schwartz, and Kelly D. Brownell. "Weight Stigmatization and Bias Reduction: Perspectives of Overweight and Obese Adults." *Health Education Research* 23, no. 2 (April 2008): 347–358.

Räikkönen, Katri, Karen A. Matthews, and Lewis H. Kuller. "The Relationship between Psychological Risk Attributes and the Metabolic Syndrome in Healthy Women: Antecedent or Consequence?" *Metabolism: Clinical and Experimental* 51, no. 12 (December 2002): 1573–1577.

Rawn, Melanie. *Playing to the Gods.* Glass Thorns series, book 5. New York: Tor, 2017.

Rippe, James M., and Theodore J. Angelopoulos. "Sugars and Health Controversies: What Does the Science Say?" *Advances in Nutrition* 6, no. 4 (July 1, 2015): 493S–503S.

Robison, Jon. "Beware the 'Cockroach Effect'—Faulty Data That Will Not Die!" LinkedIn, May 9, 2016. https://www.linkedin.com/pulse/beware-cockroach -effect-faulty-data-die-jon-robison.

Robison, Jon. "A Little Nutrition Sanity—Sugar: The Other White Powder— Rhetoric vs. Reality," LinkedIn, August 18, 2015. https://www.linkedin .com/pulse/little-nutrition-sanity-sugar-other-white-powder-rhetoric-jon -robison.

Robison, Jon, and Karen Carrier. *The Spirit and Science of Holistic Health: More Than Broccoli, Jogging, and Bottled Water . . . More Than Yoga, Herbs, and Meditation.* Bloomington, IN: AuthorHouse, 2004.

Robison, Jon, Carmen Cool, and E. Jackson. "Helping without Harming: Kids, Eating, Weight & Health." *Absolute Advantage* 7, no. 1 (2007): 2–15.

Rosenthal, Lisa, Valerie A. Earnshaw, Amy Carroll-Scott, Kathryn E. Henderson, Susan M. Peters, Catherine McCaslin, and Jeannette R. Ickovics. "Weight- and Race-Based Bullying: Health Associations among Urban Adolescents." *Journal of Health Psychology* 20, no. 4 (April 2015): 401–412.

Rothblum, Esther. "Slim Chance for Permanent Weight Loss." *Archives of Scientific Psychology* 6 (2018): 63–69.

Rothblum, Esther, and Sondra Solovay, eds. *The Fat Studies Reader.* New York: NYU Press, 2009.

Rowell, Katja, and Jenny McGlothlin. *Helping Your Child with Extreme Picky Eating.* Oakland, CA: New Harbinger Publications, 2015.

Saguy, Abigail. *What's Wrong with Fat?: The War on Obesity and Its Collateral Damage.* New York: Oxford University Press, 2013.

Salomonsen, J. "Weight Loss Does Not Prolong the Lives of Diabetes Patients." *ScienceNordic*, February 11, 2016.

Salsburg, David. *The Lady Tasting Tea: How Statistics Revolutionized Science in the Twentieth Century.* New York: Holt Paperbacks, 2002.

Santos-Longhurst, Adrienne. "Type 2 Diabetes Statistics and Facts." Healthline, September 8, 2014. https://www.healthline.com/health/type-2-diabetes /statistics.

Satter, Ellyn. *Child of Mine: Feeding with Love and Good Sense.* Rev. ed. Boulder, CO: Bull Publishing Company, 2000.

Shaw, Jacqueline, and Marika Tiggemann. "Dieting and Working Memory: Preoccupying Cognitions and the Role of the Articulatory Control Process." *British Journal of Health Psychology* 9, Pt 2 (May 2004): 175–185.

Sims, E. "Studies in Human Hyperphagia." In *Treatment and Management of Obesity*, edited by George A Bray and John E. Bethune, 28–44. Hagerstown, MD: Medical Dept., Harper & Row, 1974.

Smink, Frédérique R. E., Daphne van Hoeken, and Hans W. Hoek. "Epidemiology of Eating Disorders: Incidence, Prevalence and Mortality Rates." *Current Psychiatry Reports* 14, no. 4 (August 2012): 406–414.

Solovay, Sondra. *Tipping the Scales of Justice: Fighting Weight Based Discrimination.* Amherst, NY: Prometheus Books, 2000.

Sonneville, Kendrin R., Jerel P. Calzo, Nicholas J. Horton, Jess Haines, S. Bryn Austin, and Alison E. Field. "Body Satisfaction, Weight Gain, and Binge Eating among Overweight Adolescent Girls." *International Journal of Obesity* 36, no. 7 (July 2012): 944–949.

Stice, Eric, and Mark J. Van Ryzin. "A Prospective Test of the Temporal Sequencing of Risk Factor Emergence in the Dual Pathway Model of Eating Disorders." *Journal of Abnormal Psychology* 128, no. 2 (December 20, 2018): 119–128.

Stoner, Lee, and Jon Cornwall. "Did the American Medical Association Make the Correct Decision Classifying Obesity as a Disease?" *Australasian Medical Journal* 7, no. 11 (November 30, 2014): 462–464.

Stunkard, A., and M. McLaren-Hume. "The Results of Treatment for Obesity: A Review of the Literature and Report of a Series." *A.M.A. Archives of Internal Medicine* 103, no. 1 (January 1959): 79–85.

Stunkard, A. J., T. I. Sørensen, C. Hanis, T. W. Teasdale, R. Chakraborty, W. J. Schull, and F. Schulsinger. "An Adoption Study of Human Obesity." *New England Journal of Medicine* 314, no. 4 (January 23, 1986): 193–198.

Swenne, Ingemar, Thomas Parling, and Helena Salonen Ros. "Family-Based Intervention in Adolescent Restrictive Eating Disorders: Early Treatment Response and Low Weight Suppression Is Associated with Favourable One-Year Outcome." *BMC Psychiatry* 17, no. 333 (2017): 1–10.

Taylor, Sonya Renee. *The Body Is Not an Apology: The Power of Radical Self-Love.* Oakland, CA: Berrett-Koehler, 2018.

Tomiyama, A. Janet. "Weight Stigma Is Stressful. A Review of Evidence for the Cyclic Obesity/Weight-Based Stigma Model." *Appetite* 82 (November 2014): 8–15.

Tomiyama, A. Janet, Britt Ahlstrom, and Traci Mann. "Long-Term Effects of Dieting: Is Weight Loss Related to Health?" *Social and Personality Psychology Compass* 7, no. 12 (2013): 861–877.

Tomiyama, A. Janet, Deborah Carr, Ellen M. Granberg, Brenda Major, Eric Robinson, Angelina R. Sutin, and Alexandra Brewis. "How and Why Weight Stigma Drives the Obesity 'Epidemic' and Harms Health." *BMC Medicine* 16 (August 15, 2018): 1–6.

Tomiyama, A. Janet, Elissa S. Epel, Trissa M. McClatchey, Gina Poelke, Margaret E. Kemeny, Shannon K. McCoy, and Jennifer Daubenmier. "Associations of Weight Stigma with Cortisol and Oxidative Stress Independent of Adiposity." *Health Psychology: Official Journal of the Division of Health Psychology, American Psychological Association* 33, no. 8 (August 2014): 862–867.

Tomiyama, A. Janet, and Traci Mann. "If Shaming Reduced Obesity, There Would Be No Fat People." *Hastings Center Report* 43, no. 3 (June 2013): 4–5; discussion 9–10.

Tomiyama, A. Janet, Traci Mann, Danielle Vinas, Jeffrey M. Hunger, Jill DeJager, and Shelley E. Taylor. "Low Calorie Dieting Increases Cortisol." *Psychosomatic Medicine* 72, no. 4 (May 2010): 357–364.

Tovar, Virgie. *You Have the Right to Remain Fat.* New York: The Feminist Press at CUNY, 2018.

Tsai, Adam Gilden, and Thomas A. Wadden. "Systematic Review: An Evaluation of Major Commercial Weight Loss Programs in the United States." *Annals of Internal Medicine* 142, no. 1 (January 4, 2005): 56–66.

Tucker, Todd. *The Great Starvation Experiment: The Heroic Men Who Starved So That Millions Could Live.* Minneapolis, MN: Simon & Schuster, Inc., 2006.

Twitty, Michael. *The Cooking Gene: A Journey through African American Culinary History in the Old South.* New York: HarperCollins, 2017.

Tylka, Tracy L. "Development and Psychometric Evaluation of a Measure of Intuitive Eating." *Journal of Counseling Psychology* 53, no. 2 (April 2006): 226–240.

Tylka, Tracy L., Rachel A. Annunziato, Deb Burgard, Sigrún Daníelsdóttir, Ellen Shuman, Chad Davis, and Rachel M. Calogero. "The Weight-Inclusive versus Weight-Normative Approach to Health: Evaluating the Evidence for Prioritizing Well-Being over Weight Loss." *Journal of Obesity* 2014 (2014): 1–18.

Vartanian, Lenny R., and Jacqueline G. Shaprow. "Effects of Weight Stigma on Exercise Motivation and Behavior: A Preliminary Investigation among College-Aged Females." *Journal of Health Psychology* 13, no. 1 (January 2008): 131–138.

Vartanian, Lenny R., and Joshua M. Smyth. "Primum Non Nocere: Obesity Stigma and Public Health." *Journal of Bioethical Inquiry* 10, no. 1 (March 2013): 49–57.

Wann, Marilyn. *FAT!SO?: Because You Don't Have to Apologize for Your Size.* Berkeley, CA: Ten Speed Press, 1998.

Wansink, Brian, Lara A. Latimer, and Lizzy Pope. "'Don't Eat So Much:' How Parent Comments Relate to Female Weight Satisfaction." *Eating and Weight Disorders* 22, no. 3 (September 2017): 475–481.

Warner, Anthony. *The Angry Chef's Guide to Spotting Bullsh*t in the World of Food: Bad Science and the Truth about Healthy Eating.* 1st ed. New York: The Experiment, LLC, 2018.

West, Lindy. *Shrill: Notes from a Loud Woman.* New York: Hachette Books, 2017.

Wildman, Rachel P., Paul Muntner, Kristi Reynolds, Aileen P. McGinn, Swapnil Rajpathak, Judith Wylie-Rosett, and MaryFran R. Sowers. "The Obese without Cardiometabolic Risk Factor Clustering and the Normal Weight with Cardiometabolic Risk Factor Clustering: Prevalence and Correlates of 2 Phenotypes among the US Population (NHANES 1999–2004)." *Archives of Internal Medicine* 168, no. 15 (August 11, 2008): 1617–1624.

Wirth, M. D., C. E. Blake, J. R. Hébert, X. Sui, and S. N. Blair. "Metabolic Syndrome and Discrepancy between Actual and Self-Identified Good Weight: Aerobics Center Longitudinal Study." *Body Image* 13 (March 2015): 28–32.

Wolf, Naomi. *The Beauty Myth: How Images of Beauty Are Used against Women.* New York: Harper Collins, 1991.

Wooley, Orland W., and Susan C. Wooley. "The Beverly Hills Eating Disorder: The Mass Marketing of Anorexia Nervosa." *International Journal of Eating Disorders* 1, no. 3 (1982): 57–69.

Wrangham, Richard. *Catching Fire: How Cooking Made Us Human.* New York: Basic Books, 2010.

The Writing Group for the SEARCH for Diabetes in Youth Study. "Incidence of Diabetes in Youth in the United States." *JAMA* 297, no. 24 (June 27, 2007): 2716–2724.

Yeh, Susan. "Laws and Social Norms: Unintended Consequences of Obesity Laws." *University of Cincinnati Law Review* 81 (2013): 52.

Yoo, Jina H. "No Clear Winner: Effects of *The Biggest Loser* on the Stigmatization of Obese Persons." *Health Communication* 28, no. 3 (2013): 294–303.

Zhao, Yafu, and William Encinosa. "An Update on Hospitalizations for Eating Disorders, 1999 to 2009: Statistical Brief #120." In *Healthcare Cost and Utilization Project (HCUP) Statistical Briefs*. Rockville, MD: Agency for Healthcare Research and Quality, 2006.

Ziauddeen, Hisham, Sadaf Farooqi, and Paul Fletcher. "Obesity and the Brain: How Convincing Is the Addiction Model?" *Nature Reviews Neuroscience* 13, no. 4 (2012): 279–286.

Index

About the Author

Nancy Ellis-Ordway earned a BS from Eastern Illinois University in 1974 and an MSW from Washington University in St. Louis, Missouri, in 1979. She completed the Advanced Psychodynamic Psychotherapy program through the St. Louis Psychoanalytic Institute in 1989 while pregnant and then taking care of a new baby. After her children left for college, she returned to school and completed a PhD in Health Education and Promotion at the University of Missouri, Columbia, in 2016. She has a private practice in Jefferson City, Missouri. She has a daughter, son, son-in-law, daughter-in-law, and one grandson, so far. She lives with her husband at the edge of the woods outside Jefferson City. She intends to spend her retirement undermining the dominant paradigm.